TAI CHI CH'UAN

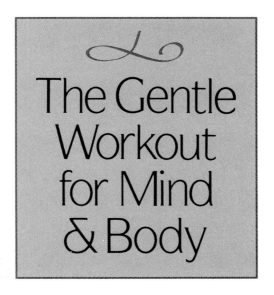

The Gentle
Workout
for Mind
& Body

*Wei Yue Sun, M.D.
& William Chen, Ph.D.*

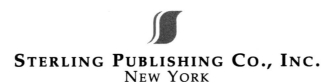

STERLING PUBLISHING CO., INC.
NEW YORK

Edited by Jeanette Green

Library of Congress Cataloging-in-Publication Data

Sun, Wei Yue.
    Tai chi ch'uan : the gentle workout for mind & body / by Wei Yue
Sun and William Chen.
        p.   cm.
    Includes index.
    ISBN 0-8069-1366-5
    1. T'ai chi ch'uan.   I. Chen, William.   II. Title.
GV504.S86   1995
613.7'148—dc20   95-17865
                                                                          CIP

                    3   5   7   9   10   8   6   4

Published by Sterling Publishing Company, Inc.
387 Park Avenue South, New York, N.Y. 10016
© 1995 by Wei Yue Sun and William Chen
Distributed in Canada by Sterling Publishing
% Canadian Manda Group, One Atlantic Avenue, Suite 105
Toronto, Ontario, Canada M6K 3E7
Distributed in Great Britain and Europe by Cassell PLC
Wellington House, 125 Strand, London WC2R 0BB, England
Distributed in Australia by Capricorn Link (Australia) Pty Ltd.
P.O. Box 6651, Baulkham Hills, Business Centre, NSW 2153, Australia
Manufactured in the United States of America
All rights reserved

Sterling ISBN 0-8069-1366-5

CONTENTS

What Is Tai Chi Ch'uan?

History

Tai chi ch'uan has been practiced for centuries in China, but its origin is uncertain. According to Chinese historical records, several tai chi ch'uan-like exercises existed before current forms of tai chi ch'uan were created.

Han Gong-yue, during the Liang reign (A.D. 502–557) of the South-North dynasty, taught the Nine Small Heaven method to the governor of the Anhui province. This physical art has been considered by some Chinese historians as the earliest pre–tai chi ch'uan exercise. About a century later, during the Tang dynasty (A.D. 618–907), Yu Fan-zi taught the physical art of Long Ch'uan, which bore similarities to the Nine Small Heaven method. In the late Tang dynasty, Li Dao-shan is credited with creating Preheaven Ch'uan, an extended form of the physical exercises taught by his two predecessors, Han Gong-yue and Yu Fan-zi. Later, Yan Li-heng created the Postheaven method, which is similar to the tai chi ch'uan practiced today.

Zhang San-feng is usually credited as the founder of tai chi ch'uan in the 1500s. He taught a form of physical and martial art based on different pre–tai chi ch'uan exercises. Soon after that, tai chi ch'uan was divided into northern and southern branches. Most tai chi ch'uan practiced today comes from the northern branch and has been modified and combined with other martial arts.

Through the centuries, the northern branch was in turn divided into additional branches, like the Chen, Yang, Wu, and Sun styles. These different styles or branches are popularly taught in different regions of China. Although these styles all have health benefits, most remain long and complicated and too difficult to learn without an instructor.

The Chinese National Physical Education Administration (CNPEA), realizing the need of the growing number of people wanting to learn tai chi ch'uan, convened the first national workshop in 1970 in Beijing, where masters of different styles of tai chi ch'uan came from all over China to work together. With the aid of these experts, the CNPEA developed the first form of tai chi ch'uan to combine the different regional styles. They also made tai chi ch'uan easy to learn. This Simplified Tai Chi Ch'uan has 24 forms and is sometimes referred to as Beijing Short-Form Tai Chi Ch'uan.

Simplified or Beijing Short-Form Tai Chi Ch'uan, credited by the CNPEA, was taught across China from 1970 to 1988. It was thought to be a practical and simple way to learn the physical art. But many experts found drawbacks to the method. They thought it was not comprehensive enough to represent the different styles of tai chi ch'uan. This simplified method also focused more on physical movement while ignoring the elements of breathing, eye movement, and mental concentration integral to most martial arts. And this simplified method was also less useful for self-defense.

So, CNPEA convened another national workshop in 1988, inviting experts of the different styles to Anhui to create a more comprehensive and beneficial tai chi ch'uan. From this workshop New Style Tai Chi Ch'uan was developed, which expanded the Beijing Short-Form and incorporated additional movements from different regional styles of tai chi ch'uan. New Style Tai Chi Ch'uan emphasizes breathing, eye movement, and mental concentration, elements left out of the 1970 version.

The art of tai chi ch'uan was thought to have been created from observations of natural phenomena, with attention to the physiological needs of the human nervous system. This art represents the accumulated wisdom and expresses the essence of the Chinese martial arts. Its postures and movements remain free, smooth, and natural. Although the movements appear light or soft, they can exert a force that's extremely hard and strong. That's why tai chi ch'uan training is such an admired type of physical exercise and meditation that millions of people practice to develop and draw on their potential inner energies. For many practitioners, it represents the best of the martial arts. And through the centuries, it has remained an invaluable treasure of Chinese culture.

Theory

Tai chi ch'uan has been described as an exercise, dance, religious ritual, philosophy of life, method of achieving mental peace and relaxation. This ancient Chinese sport, sometimes called shadow boxing, is a philosophical exercise or art with the aim of harmonizing the mind and the body. Its relaxed, smooth, and graceful movements make it suitable for children as well as the elderly and for people in all physical conditions, except for those with severe physical handicaps.

The Chinese word *tai* means the "ultimate supreme" and the word *chi* means the "ridgepole of a house." Put together, the words *tai chi* create the image of a great ridgepole capable of supporting and nurturing all things in the universe. Some Chinese people have even believed that mental and physical well-being depends on tai chi, seen as the source of life. The noun *ch'uan* means "an exercise involving the fists and boxing," and the verb *ch'uan* means "to clasp." So, when we combine all three Chinese words within the context of Chinese philosophy, *tai chi ch'uan* suggests a type of boxing exercise that attempts to clasp or hold in harmony the great yin and yang energies residing inside an individual woman or man.

The art of tai chi ch'uan necessarily rests on yin and yang, dual forces seen as complementary opposites thought to permeate the universe. In Chinese philosophy, tai chi ch'uan derives its vital energies, indeed even its very physical and mental constitution, as do all things in the universe, from yin and yang. To understand tai chi ch'uan's benefits, let's look at the traditional interplay of yin and yang elements found in all facets of exercise.

Yin and yang are alternating forces, negative and positive, that flow through all things in nature. They're treated as polarities—earth and heaven, moon and sun, woman and man, softness and firmness, quiescence and motion. The human body contains this polarity as well, since we stand erect, with a trunk acting as an axis around which the body rotates. When the right hand pushes forward, the left hand naturally draws back. As we step forward with the right foot, the left foot glides back.

According to traditional Chinese theory, yin (passive) and yang (active) are not separate entities but two faces of the same coin, and some portion of the one exists in the other. Tai chi ch'uan routines consist of these passive and active elements—stillness and movement, rest and motion, curved and straight, contraction and expansion, exhalation and inhalation, closed and open, left and right, backwards and forward, settling and floating.

In Chinese culture, balanced yin and yang energies are thought vital for good health, and it's thought that people become sick when this balance is broken. The circular movements of tai chi ch'uan mirror this important balance. A yang form always follows a yin form and vice versa. A forward movement or side movement is always followed by a movement backwards or to the other side. These physical activities also necessarily involve internal work, since mind and body participate in the same energies.

Tai Chi Ch'uan's Benefits

Health Benefits

For older people, tai chi ch'uan can be highly recommended as a form of exercise. It's safe, effective, and invigorating. These movements aren't too strenuous even for many people in poor health, and they can be performed at any speed for any chosen length of time. A single form like "Parting the Wild Horse's Mane, Left" (35) uses every part of the body and helps develop balance and coordination. Tai chi ch'uan does not demand strenuous cardiovascular output; so, it is an ideal exercise for cardiac patients or for others who have not been physically active. These exercises improve flexibility, strength, and balance safely for such patients.

The slow, supple movements of tai chi ch'uan facilitate deep breathing, making it more rhythmic and easy. These movements also greatly improve circulation, supplying blood to all organs of the body. And improved circulation means improved efficiency of the body in receiving oxygen and nutrients.

While many Chinese people practice tai chi ch'uan to socialize and keep fit, they also recognize its many positive attributes. Tai chi ch'uan improves functioning of the neurological, cardiovascular, gastrointestinal, and skeletal systems. Lung capacity increases, digestion improves, muscles strengthen, and joints and limbs become stronger and more flexible.

Effects on Heart and Blood Pressure

Western health professionals have begun to recognize how tai chi ch'uan can aid in preventing heart disease, one of the chief causes of death in the Western world. Its practice can help regulate blood pressure and condition and strengthen the heart.

Since tai chi ch'uan is a gentle, relaxing form of exercise, it's also recommended as relaxation therapy for the chronically ill. Since its movements are slow and graceful, they can be performed without nervous tension. This allows the blood, and the body's vital energies, to circulate freely. Tai chi ch'uan has been widely used to improve the cardiovascular system. It can reduce high blood pressure without medication. The practice also helps teach people to conserve energy, reduce stress, and relax in a dynamic way. These are important benefits for coronary heart disease patients who need to lower their blood pressure, learn relaxation, tone muscles without strain, and not exert themselves in performing routine tasks.

In a study at the Beijing Research Institute, Professor Qu Mianya compared the general health of 32 people who practiced tai chi ch'uan with that of 56 others who did not practice it. The subjects, ages 50 to 89, were all monitored under the same conditions. Only 28 percent of tai chi ch'uan practitioners had abnormal electrocardiograms (EKGs), while about 41 percent of the nonpractitioners had abnormal EKGs. The average blood pressure of tai chi ch'uan practitioners was 134/81 while that of nonpractitioners was 155/83. Arteriosclerosis was present in about 40 percent of the practitioners compared with 46 percent of the nonpractitioners.

In our own Florida pilot study of people 50 and older, 23 participants received 4 months' instruction in this simple form of tai chi ch'uan and were asked to practice daily at home for 9 months following instruction. At the end of the 9-month period, these participants' blood pressure improved compared with our 13 control subjects.

Tai chi ch'uan appears to benefit healthy people as well as those with high blood pressure or heart conditions.

Effects on Stress Management

Tai chi ch'uan helps develop balance and coordination while enhancing emotional well-being and mental health. The traditional goals of tai chi ch'uan are to strengthen the body, exercise internal organs, and develop the mind. In the mind-body coordination and mental concentration necessary for this exercise, you can practice a kind of holistic meditation with the goals of self-awareness, relaxation, mental organization, personal direction, dynamic thinking, and enhanced energy. During this meditation the body remains completely relaxed. In some styles of tai chi ch'uan mental imagery enhances the basic structure of the forms.

Since the mind and body are linked, tai chi ch'uan, which attends to the needs of both, is a complete exercise. Its practice engages the whole person and can improve both physical and mental functioning. A tranquil mind is necessary for a relaxed body. Tai chi ch'uan's slow, calming movements aid concentration and mental calm since the mind focuses on the exercise. With regular practice your mind will be less likely to wander, and your memory may improve since you need to remember each movement and form in the sequence. Tai chi ch'uan can facilitate the flow of mental and emotional processes. It can even help sharpen your thinking as it soothes and softens your responses in traditional yin and yang fashion. Since it successfully reduces tension, ill temper may disappear. Its soft, repetitive movements can provide a feeling of contentment and intellectual calm within self-discovery.

Tai chi ch'uan also aids posture or body alignment, which will reduce physical stress and allow good circulation. It permits dynamic relaxation of both mind and body.

Effects on Joint Flexibility

The practice of tai chi ch'uan improves the body's flexibility. These exercises increase the range of motion of the joints while strengthening them and improving balance. They enhance body awareness, both internally and externally. They also involve larger body dynamics, since the spiral movements of these exercises follow the body's anatomical structure.

Although tai chi ch'uan appears slow and easy, much is taking place. One of tai chi ch'uan's virtues is that it uses the entire body—shoulders, elbows, palms, fingers, abdomen, hips, buttocks, legs, knees, sides and soles of the feet, toes, and eyes. The isometric work of holding a muscle in tension, then relaxing it, rapidly improves muscle tone. Although these movements are gentle, they productively stimulate and exercise muscles. Illnesses that limit flexibility, like arthritis, rheumatism, lumbago, sciatica, and multiple sclerosis, can be safely treated with tai chi ch'uan.

These slow, gentle exercises require use of large muscle masses. The circular movements gently rotate the body through the horizontal axis of the joints. These exercises naturally require the body to move as a whole rather than as an aggregate of individual muscles and limbs. Many other forms of "spot" exercises isolate muscles like those in the abdomen or the calves.

Tai chi ch'uan works on the body as a whole. With tai chi ch'uan, you initiate movement from the trunk of the body, and the body's momentum, as when walking, is reflected in the hands. So, the whole body becomes involved in the exercise.

These exercises, characterized by spiral and diagonal patterns of movement, seem a natural extension of the spiral and rotary nature of the bones, joints, and ligaments. This type of motion is in harmony with the anatomical alignment of the muscles from origin to insertion and with the structure of individual muscles.

Muscles, tendons, ligaments, and cartilage all have a spiral structure. Even bones rotate with the aid of these structures. So, these spiral movements made in the direction of the muscle fibers help improve joint and muscle capabilities. These exercises also use horizontal movements, which stimulate and increase the motion of synovial fluid through the joints, thereby improving nutrition for the cartilage.

In a Canadian study, subjects age 24 to 35 practicing tai chi ch'uan for an average of 5 years had flexibility scores around the 90th percentile for the Canadian population. In another study of subjects age 50 to 89, 77.4 percent could touch their toes while only 16.6 percent of control subjects, who did not practice tai chi ch'uan, could do so. In yet another study, tai chi ch'uan was found to increase shoulder flexion and extension by 26.8 degrees in just 12 weeks of practice in a group of people age 60 to 74.

For the elderly, increased flexibility may lead to increased independence, greater self-reliance, and improved quality of life. Flexibility in turn improves mobility and maneuverability, making older people less vulnerable to accident and injury.

Concentration and Calm

It's important to have a calm disposition when assuming the starting position for a given form or movement. Do not let your thoughts ramble. Clear your mind so that you become peaceful, placid, and undistracted. Make sure every part of your body is correctly aligned, and ask yourself if you feel relaxed. In this preparatory stage, the mind may seem to float inside the body. Observe your body in descending order—head, throat, shoulders, arms, hands, chest, stomach, legs, and feet. Then observe your feet, legs, buttocks, waist, back, neck, and head in reverse, ascending, order. Be sure to check this circular route again and again, adjusting any incorrect posture and immediately relaxing any stiffness you feel in the limbs.

Most of us are in the habit of maintaining tension in different parts of the body that is difficult to dispel. When the mind concentrates passively, it helps us relax, but when our attention falters, these physical tensions (that we're often unaware of) may return. That's why we need to check the different parts of the body, adjust ourselves, and form the new habit of feeling relaxed and peaceful.

Dantian and Chi During all tai chi ch'uan movements, your mind should concentrate on the *dantian* (the center of your body), a spot 2 or 3 inches (5 to 7.5 cm) below the navel, or on *chi*, the flow of energy, to different body parts in coordination with the particular forms and movements.

Coordination

Tai chi ch'uan is an exercise for the whole person rather than a series of spot exercises for specific limbs or other body parts. Since this exercise combines inner energy with physical movement, it helps coordinate or harmonize both body and mind.

To achieve comfortable coordination, remember that the whole body moves in tai chi ch'uan as one entity. So, the movement of the arms should be in harmony with a corresponding movement of the legs. Make the dantian the center from which all movements begin and flow to the extremities. Be sure to concentrate on the dantian from the very first time you learn and practice tai chi ch'uan.

Breathing

Allow your movements to guide your breathing, thereby coordinating your mind and breath with each movement in the sequence of forms. One inhalation should naturally be followed by one exhalation. Inhale deeply and calmly into the center of your body through your nose, and guide your breathing with your mind by concentrating on this center, the dantian. Exhale with a deep and calm breath out of the dantian through the mouth, using the motion of your mind from the body's center to the different body parts coordinated with the particular tai chi ch'uan movements.

Weight Shifting

Weight distribution and firm footing are

important since they affect how you change positions. When practicing tai chi ch'uan you need to shift your weight from one foot to another except for a few beginning and closing movements. Shift your weight in a flowing motion from emptiness to fullness in one leg and fullness to emptiness in the other. If you do not achieve this, stable footing won't be possible, your body alignment will be shaky, and you'll look and feel awkward. Maintain good balance when shifting and distributing your weight to assure calm and even movements of your arms and legs.

Body Alignment

Head　Hold the head naturally straight. *Bai-hui*, the center of the top of the head, is according to Chinese medicine an important major nerve center that regulates hundreds of other auxiliary nerve centers. When the *bai-hui* functions well, we feel alert, relaxed, and comfortable. Keeping your head naturally straight will increase the flow of inner energy into it and in turn increase blood circulation.

Eyelids　The upper and lower eyelids need to relax along with all your facial muscles. With relaxed eyelids, you can fully concentrate and not be distracted by outside interferences.

Tongue　The tip of the tongue should touch the upper palate and the upper teeth should touch the lower teeth gently. In a relaxed position, the tip of the tongue curls up slightly, touching the upper palate without pressure. This helps connect the head with the body and allows inner energy to flow freely between the head and the body.

Neck　Since most major nerves and blood vessels run through the neck vertically, when the neck is not upright and relaxed, circulation becomes blocked and this affects the functioning of the whole body. That's why it's important to keep the neck upright and relaxed.

Shoulders　Allow your shoulders to relax and hang down naturally. The shoulder joint holds the scapula and clavicle together. When the triangular muscles of the shoulder and the back and chest muscles are stimulated, they sometimes contract and cause the shoulders to rise, making hand movements sluggish. By keeping your shoulders down, you can help nearby muscles relax naturally so that your upper body can move freely and easily.

Throat and Chest　Keep the upper throat hidden (pull your chin in) so that your chest will be relaxed and your inner energy can flow naturally, increasing your circulation.

Spine and Waist　Keep the spine upright and relax the waist. Remember that the spine supports the whole body and the waist governs movement of the limbs as well as other physical activities. When the spine is not upright, the posture you assume will be incorrect, and if you don't relax the waist, your whole body will not be able to move freely. When your waist is relaxed, the joints in your back become loose, allowing your inner energy to gather at the dantian. And that means strength will reach from the dantian through your arms and legs, the lower body will become stable, and the arms will maneuver freely. This permits the upper and lower body to operate in harmony.

Buttocks　Completely relax the buttocks and keep them slightly closed inward. This aids inner energy flow through the dantian to your legs and from your legs back to the dantian, increasing circulation.

Feet As the foundation of the body, the feet support every posture and movement. Keep them parallel to balance your upper body and to prevent it from inclining forward or backwards or making you lose your balance. When your legs are parallel, the space in your groin (between your abdomen and upper thighs) becomes round. When your knees close inward, your legs form an arch and produce a kind of circular thrust of strength.

Arms Arm movement should be circular. When your back is slightly arched, your shoulders and elbows dipped, and your wrists stretched, both arms can move in a circular way. The space between the middle fingers of both hands seems linked by an imaginary line so that both arms appear to complete a circle. During these exercises, all movements must describe a circle. You'll be creating large and small circles, larger circles will contain small ones, and small circles will be mixed with large circles. This allows energy to travel through both arms.

HOW NEW STYLE TAI CHI CH'UAN DIFFERS FROM OTHER STYLES

Most tai chi ch'uan books focus on physical movement and teach beginners to remember simply the sequences of forms and movements. Without internal mental exercise or concentration, tai chi ch'uan's benefits do not greatly differ from other types of exercise, like running, biking, and weight-lifting. New Style Tai Chi Ch'uan, presented in this book, combines physical movement with eye movement, breathing, mental exercise, and *chi*, energy flow. We also include self-defense applications for each movement.

Properly practiced, New Style Tai Chi Ch'uan increases internal energies and does not simply work large muscle groups, say of the legs and arms, or isolated muscles. Chi flows from mental exercise and this mental concentration follows eye movement. Breathing is also important to these movements. When you inhale, you can store your energy in the dantian guided by mental exercise. You can then move this energy out to your hands and feet by exhaling. In this way, physical movement, mental exercise, eye movement, and breathing work together to perform the whole tai chi ch'uan movement within a given form.

Eye Movement

In New Style Tai Chi Ch'uan, whenever you use your arm, hand, palm, foot, or heel to protect yourself or attack an opponent, you must use your eyes to monitor the part of your body you want to use as well as to observe your opponent.

Breathing

Continue breathing in the whole tai chi ch'uan sequence, with deep exhalation following each deep inhalation for each movement. This is how you can store your energy or chi and direct it throughout your whole body or to the part of your body you need to use for exercise or self-defense.

Mental Exercise

In addition to physical exercise, tai chi ch'uan exercises the mind, thereby improving the overall well-being of the practitioner. Adopt passive concentration when you assume each form. Concentrating on the body's movements will aid mental concentration. First, focus mental energy on the dantian, where you've stored your energy, and when you focus mental energy on a body part needed for movement, chi will automatically flow into that part.

Self-Defense

The primary objective of tai chi ch'uan is relaxation and energy enhancement, but it can also be used for self-defense. For example, when assuming form (5) "Right Press" (*You An*), the movement can be changed to repel an attack from the left and right sides. But tai chi ch'uan practitioners should not be preoccupied with self-defense. As you grow very familiar with each movement, you will be able to naturally transform it or continue each movement into self-defense use. Your body will follow your mind's command to defend

yourself should you find yourself in a dangerous situation.

But knowing that self-defense can be an important extension of basic tai chi ch'uan movements will help you perfect or perform each correctly since you will understand its purpose. So, learning that the purpose of moving your right hand and palm is to protect your face from attack from the right side, this self-defense movement becomes easier to learn. And it helps you naturally move your right hand and palm correctly.

Combining Breathing, Mental Exercise, and Self-Defense

It is important to integrate your concentration and inner energy when practicing tai chi ch'uan since various distractions often interfere. Over time this can cause you to misdirect your vital activities.

In tai chi ch'uan you learn to keep the mind at rest in a placid state, adjust body alignment, and regularize breathing to maximize the benefit of tai chi ch'uan's inner energy. When practicing tai chi ch'uan forms, remember to keep your concentration on the dantian. In this way, Taoism also teaches people to dispense with distractions and excitement.

Inner energy refers to vital life activities, linking the limbs with internal organs that regulate bodily functions and maintain life. When the body has insufficient inner energy and your energy flow is not smooth, it's likely to malfunction. If you block the flow of inner energy within the body, illness often follows. Without inner energy, life ceases to exist.

Integrating your concentration with your inner energy means that you consciously control breathing to stimulate specific body parts. To harmonize your mind with breathing, mentally concentrate on the dantian and be aware of the energy coming in from the outside that you can store in the dantian. At the same time, inhale deeply through your nose. While exhaling through your mouth, visualize inner energy coming from the dantian and flowing to different body parts according to the needs of different tai chi ch'uan movements. This inner energy flow allows you to use the particular body part, like the palms and arms, both to protect yourself and attack an opponent.

Comprehensive

New Style Tai Chi Ch'uan is more comprehensive than most versions of tai chi ch'uan. It features a greater variety of movements of fists, palms, hands, arms, and feet than other styles, which tend to repeat the same forms and movements often.

Elegant

New Style Tai Chi Ch'uan movements are elegant and continuous, since one step flows into the next within a movement and within a form and within a whole sequence of forms without stopping. So, hand and feet movements are always continuous and smooth, almost like dance.

Easy to Learn

Since New Style Tai Chi Ch'uan is based on Simplified Tai Chi Ch'uan, many movements are similar. If you have already prac-

ticed Simplified Tai Chi Ch'uan, this Yang Style will be especially easy for you to learn. New Style has the advantage of being relatively short, simple, and comprehensive. With only 78 forms, it avoids the complexity of the Yang style of Tai Chi Ch'uan with its 150 forms.

How to Practice

It's best to use this book in conjunction with a class on tai chi ch'uan, since an instructor or master will be able to help you with correct positioning. But this book contains all essentials.

New Style Tai Chi Ch'uan has five sequences of fifteen or more forms for each with a total of 78 forms. The Chinese name, for each form, transliterated from Mandarin, appears under the English name. Individual forms, like (17) "Parting the Wild Horse's Mane," have in turn one or more movements. Photos show each movement for a given form, and arrows within the photos indicate the direction of the next movement. Following each movement in the text is a description of what to do with your eyes, how to breathe properly, what your mind should concentrate on, and how to tailor the movement for self-defense.

Once you've learned all the elements of each sequence, it will take about 20 to 30 minutes to practice. Be sure to practice sequences in appropriate order (1–15 should be followed by 16–30, etc.), since each movement, form, and sequence is designed to flow into another. Ideally, you should practice all 78 forms (five sequences) for a good overall workout, but you can stop at the end of a given sequence if you have limited time.

New Style Tai Chi Ch'uan Sequences

❁

First Sequence (1–15)

(1) Preparation
Yu Bei Shi

Movement: Shift your weight completely onto your right leg. Raise the left foot and place it to the left sideways at about shoulder width, with your toes pointing directly ahead, and rest your weight on it. At the same time, bend your elbows slightly outward with the palms facing backwards. Both feet should now point directly ahead. Your weight should be centered between the two legs, and the distance between your feet equal to the distance between your shoulders. The shoulders should always be slumped, the chest depressed, and the tongue should rest against the hard palate with the mouth lightly closed. Your back should be as straight as possible. Relax the entire body completely. It's only then that chi can sink to the dantian. (See photo 1. Remember, arrows in photos indicate the direction of the next movement.)

Eyes: Look forward.

Breathing: Inhale, then exhale.

Mind: Concentrate on the dantian. p99.

Self-defense: Store energy (chi) for self-defense.

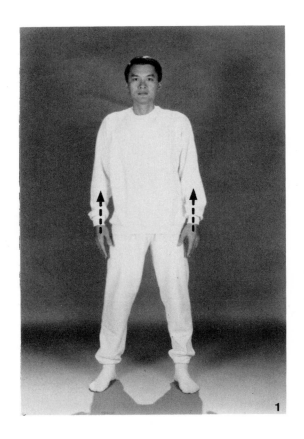

(2) Beginning
Qi Shi

Movement 1: Gradually raise the arms forward and upward to shoulder height with wrists bent, facing up, and fingers hanging down. Slowly extend the fingers so that they point forward. (See photo 2.)

Eyes: Look forward.

Breathing: Inhale.

Mind: Concentrate on the dantian.

Self-defense: Use all ten fingers to hit an opponent's eyes when he or she closes in on you.

Movement 2: Bend the elbows slightly, and allow the hands to be drawn back toward the upper chest. Lower the elbows slightly downward as you raise your fingers slightly upward. Slowly lower your hands until they are below the hip joints with palms facing backwards. Bend the elbows slightly outward and let the fingers hang downward. (See photo 3.)

Eyes: Look forward.

Breathing: Exhale.

Mind: Concentrate on the dantian.

Self-defense: Put more chi on your hands and palms.

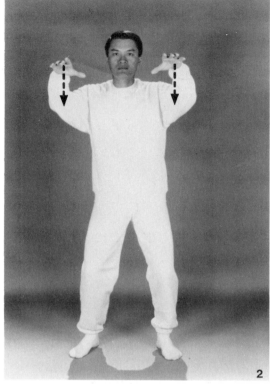

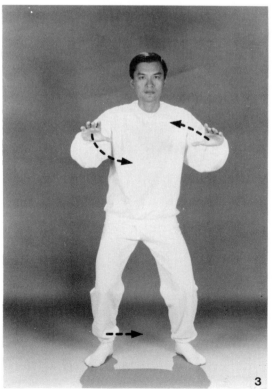

(3) White Crane Spreading Wings
Bai He Liang Chi

Movement 1: Shift your weight to your left foot and put your left hand at the height of your throat with your palm down and elbow bent. Move your right hand near the left side of your waist with the palm upward. This posture resembles holding a ball in your hands on the left side of your body. (See photo 4.)

Eyes: Follow your left hand.

Breathing: Inhale.

Mind: Concentrate on the dantian.

Self-defense: Put more chi on both hands and palms.

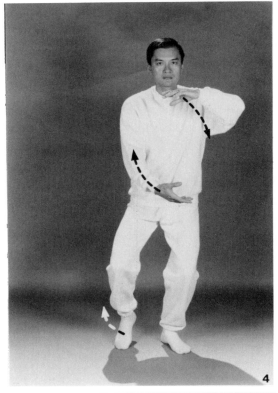

Movement 2: Shift all your weight to your right foot, allowing the left heel to rise slightly with the toes remaining on the ground. Raise your right arm, tracing a large clockwise circle through 180 degrees until your right elbow hangs at the level of your chin and your right hand (palm forward, fingers pointing upward) is above your head. Lower your left arm until the hand rests beside your left hip joint, the palm facing down. (See photo 5.)

Eyes: Follow your right hand.

Breathing: Exhale.

Mind: Direct energy from the dantian to your right arm and hand.

Self-defense: Use your right hand and palm to protect yourself against an opponent's attack on your right side. At the same time, use your left hand and palm to block your left side in case an opponent tries to kick you on that side.

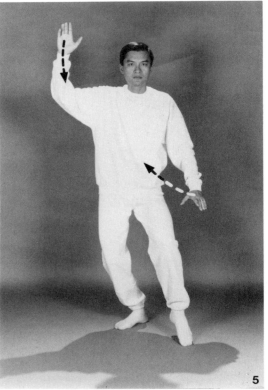

(4) Brush Left Knee and Twist Step
Zuo Lou Xi Ao Bu

Movement 1: The right hand circles upward, downward, backwards, and upward, returning to the right side of your head. At the same time, the left hand circles clockwise, backwards, upward, and forward to the right ear. This palm should face outward and be slightly inclined downward with your elbow bent. (See photo 6.)

Eyes: Look forward.

Breathing: Inhale.

Mind: Concentrate on the dantian.

Self-defense: Use your right hand and arm and your left hand and arm to protect yourself from a frontal attack.

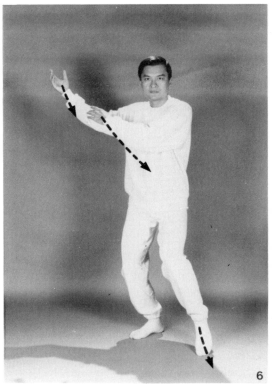

Movement 2: Turn the torso slightly to the left, and take a big step forward with the left foot, with your heel touching the ground first. Brush the left knee with the left hand, palm backwards, bringing it to rest beside the left thigh. Begin shifting your body weight to the left foot, and curve the right foot slightly inward, turning on the heel. Push your right hand forward, with the elbow slightly bent. (See photo 7.)

Eyes: Follow your right hand.

Breathing: Exhale.

Mind: Visualize energy coming from the dantian through your right arm to your right hand.

Self-defense: Use your left hand and palm to protect your left knee from an opponent's kick, and use your right hand and palm to attack an opponent in front of you.

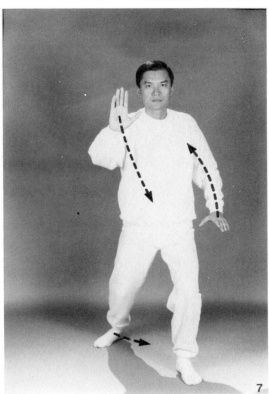

(5) Right Press
You An

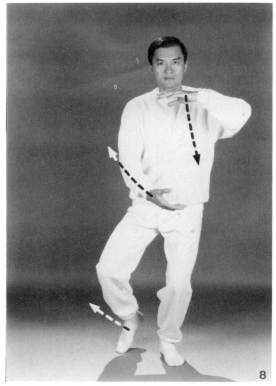

Movement 1: Shift weight onto your left leg, draw your right foot to the side of your left foot and rest the toes on the floor. Turn the body slightly to the left, assume a ball-holding gesture in front of the left side of your chest, with the left hand on top. (See photo 8.)

Eyes: Watch your left hand.

Breathing: Inhale.

Mind: Concentrate on your dantian.

Self-defense: Put more chi on both hands and palms.

Movement 2: Turn your torso to the right. Take a step forward with your right foot, and shift your weight gradually to your right. Turn your torso a bit further to the right, and bend your right leg to form a bow step with the left leg naturally straightened. Meanwhile, push out the rounded right forearm at shoulder level with palm facing inward. Drop the left hand slowly to the side of the left hip, with the palm facing downward and fingers pointing forward. (See photo 9.)

Eyes: Follow your right hand.

Breathing: Exhale.

Mind: Visualize energy coming from the dantian through your right arm to your right hand.

Self-defense: Use your right hand and arm to protect yourself from an opponent's attack from your right side.

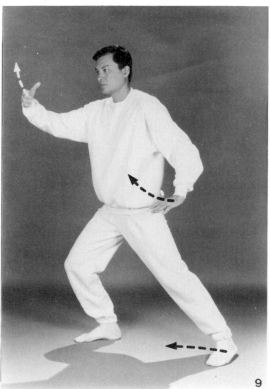

(6) Left Single Whip
Zuo Dan Bian

Movement 1: Shift your weight gradually to the left foot, turn your torso to the left, and swivel on your right heel until it faces left. As your weight shifts back to the right leg, allow the body to turn to the right slightly, and as the elbow bends, withdraw the right arm. Allow your fingers to point downward and to close together at the fingertips, forming a hook near the right armpit. (See photo 10.)

Eyes: Follow your right hand.

Breathing: Inhale.

Mind: Concentrate on your dantian.

Self-defense: Use your right hand and palm to protect yourself when an opponent closes in on your right side.

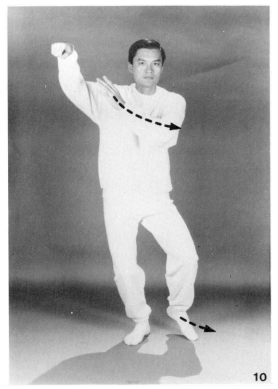

Movement 2: As the trunk turns toward the left, take a wide step to the left with the left foot. First set the heel down, then the toes, which point left. Shift your weight to the left leg. The left heel should not be directly in front of the right heel but on as wide a diagonal position as you can comfortably manage. Gradually shift the body weight to your left leg, bending the leg at the knee; at the same time, turn the left palm outward with the arm slightly bent. (See photo 11.)

Eyes: Follow your left hand.

Breathing: Exhale.

Mind: Visualize energy coming from the dantian through your left arm to your left hand.

Self-defense: Use your left hand and palm to attack an opponent on your left side.

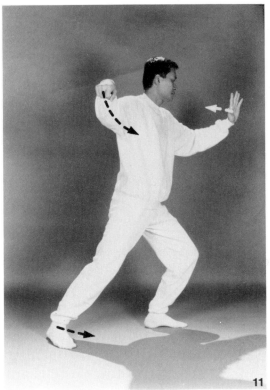

(7) Playing the Guitar and Press Right Hand
You Shou Hui Pi Pa

Movement 1: Pick up your right foot, and move it close to your left foot. Set it down and shift your entire body weight to your right foot. Shift your left foot slightly sideways to the right, and touch the ground with the heel only, in line with the right heel. At the same time, bring your right hand along in a backward arc, with your palm facing left, and bring it opposite your left elbow, raising your left hand with the palm facing right so that your fingers are in line with your mouth. Your elbow should be slightly bent and your fingers point forward. This position simulates playing a guitar. (See photo 12).

Eyes: Follow your left hand.

Breathing: Inhale.

Mind: Concentrate on your dantian.

Self-defense: Use both hands and palms to protect the upper half of your body from a frontal attack.

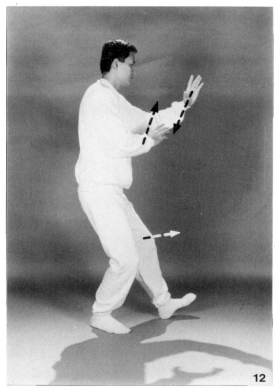

Movement 2: Move your left foot forward a step, shift your weight to it, bending the left knee slightly. Draw your left hand backwards and extend your right hand forward until your left hand is near your abdomen with your palm up and your right hand in front, over your left hand with palm forward and your elbow slightly bent. (See photo 13.)

Eyes: Follow your right hand.

Breathing: Exhale.

Mind: Visualize energy coming from the dantian through your right arm to your right hand.

Self-defense: Use your right hand to attack an opponent in front of you. At the same time, use your left hand to protect your front.

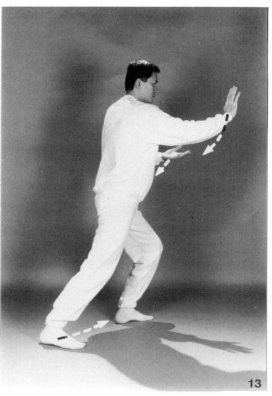

(8) Grasp the Bird's Tail, Right
You Lan Jiao Wei

Movement 1: Move your right foot close to your left foot. Turn your torso left slightly while pulling both hands down, drawing an arc in front of the left side of the abdomen, finishing with your left hand extended sideways at shoulder level, palm up, and the right forearm lying across your chest, palm turned inward. (See photo 14.)

Eyes: Follow your right hand.

Breathing: Inhale.

Mind: Concentrate on your dantian.

Self-defense: Use both arms, hands, and palms to grasp an opponent's hand and pull it to your left side.

Movement 2: Extend your right foot forward a step, shifting your weight to the right leg. Turn the torso slightly to the right. Bend your left arm and place the left hand inside your right wrist. Turn the torso a little further to the right, and press both hands slowly forward with the left palm facing forward, the right palm inward, and the right arm rounded. (See photo 15.)

Eyes: Follow both hands.

Breathing: Exhale.

Mind: Visualize energy coming from the dantian through both arms to both hands.

Self-defense: Use both hands and palms to hit your opponent's chest in front of you.

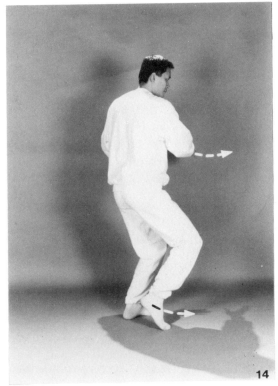

14

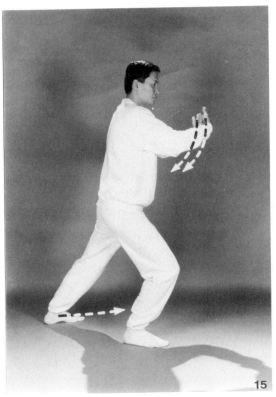

15

(9) Grasp the Bird's Tail, Left
Zuo Lan Jiao Wei

Movement 1: Move your left foot, closing to your right foot. Turn your torso to the right slightly while pulling both hands down in so that you draw an arc in front of the right side of the abdomen. Finish with your right hand extended sideways at shoulder level, palm up, and your left forearm lying across the chest, palm turned inward. (See photo 16.)

Eyes: Follow your left hand.

Breathing: Inhale.

Mind: Concentrate on your dantian.

Self-defense: Use both arms, hands, and palms to grasp your opponent's hand and pull it to your right side.

Movement 2: Extend your left foot forward a step, shifting weight to the left leg. Turn the torso slightly to the left. Bend your right arm and place your right hand inside your left wrist. Turn the torso a little further to the left, and press both hands slowly forward with the right palm facing forward, the left palm inward, and the left arm rounded. (See photo 17.)

Eyes: Follow both hands.

Breathing: Exhale.

Mind: Visualize energy coming from the dantian through both arms to both hands.

Self-defense: Use both hands and palms to hit your opponent's chest in front of you.

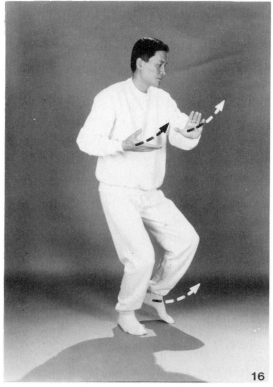

16

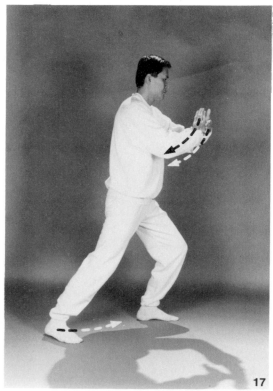

17

(10) Grasp the Bird's Tail, Right
You Lan Jiao Wei

Movement 1: Move your right foot close to your left foot. Turn your torso to the left slightly while pulling both hands down so that you draw an arc before your abdomen, finishing with the left hand extended sideways at shoulder level, palm up, and the right forearm lying across your chest, with palm turned inward. (See photo 18.)

Eyes: Follow your right hand.

Breathing: Inhale.

Mind: Concentrate on your dantian.

Self-defense: Use both arms, hands, and palms to grasp your opponent's hand and pull it to your left side.

Movement 2: Extend your right foot forward a step, shift weight to the right leg. Turn your torso slightly to the right. Bend your left arm and place your left hand inside your right wrist. Turn your torso a little further to the right, and press both hands slowly forward, with the left palm facing forward, the right palm inward, and the right arm rounded. (See photo 19.)

Eyes: Follow both hands.

Breathing: Exhale.

Mind: Visualize energy coming from the dantian through both arms to both hands.

Self-defense: Use both hands and palms in front of you to hit your opponent's chest.

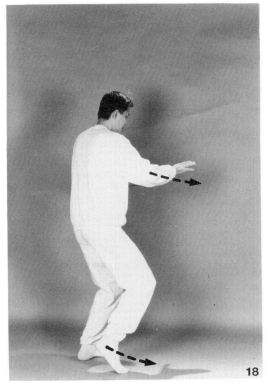

18

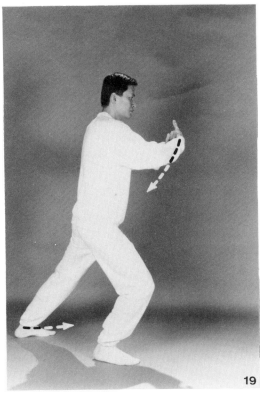

19

(11) Deflect Downward, Parry
Ban Lan Chui

Movement 1: Move your left foot close to your right foot. Simultaneously with your body, turn slightly left, as your left hand circles downward toward your right side, and then, with fingers clenched into a fist, moves past the abdomen to beside your right ribs with knuckles up. (See photo 20.)

Eyes: Follow your left hand.

Breathing: Inhale.

Mind: Concentrate on dantian.

Self-defense: Use your left arm, hand, and fist to attack an opponent in front of you.

Movement 2: Extend your left foot a step forward, and shift your weight slowly to the left leg. Turn your body left, thrust your left fist upward and forward in front of your chest, with knuckles turned down. Press your right hand against your left wrist. (See photo 21.)

Eyes: Follow your left hand.

Breathing: Exhale.

Mind: Visualize energy coming from the dantian through your left arm to your left fist.

Self-defense: Use your left arm, hand, and fist to attack an opponent in front of you.

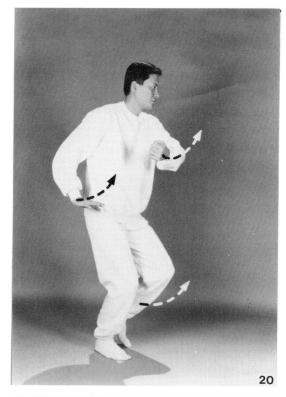

20

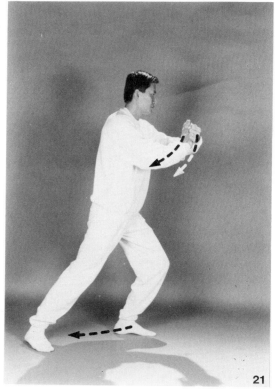

21

(12) Parting the Wild Horse's Mane, Left
Zuo Yei Ma Fen Zong

Movement 1: Turn your torso slightly to the right, and shift your weight slowly to the right leg. At the same time, bring your right hand sideways up to shoulder level, with your palm facing downward, while your left palm is turned upward. Make a ball-holding gesture in front of the right side of your chest, with your right hand on top. (See photo 22.)

Eyes: Watch your right hand.

Breathing: Inhale.

Mind: Concentrate on the dantian.

Self-defense: Put more chi on both hands and palms.

Movement 2: Step forward with your left foot. Turn the torso a bit further to the left and bend your left leg to form a bow step with your right leg naturally straightened. Shift your weight slowly to the left leg. Meanwhile, push out the rounded left forearm at shoulder level with your palm facing inward. Drop your right hand slowly to the side of your right hip, with the palm facing downward and fingers pointing forward. (See photo 23.)

Eyes: Follow the left hand.

Breathing: Exhale.

Mind: Visualize energy coming from the dantian through your left arm to the left hand.

Self-defense: Use your left arm, hand, and palm to protect yourself from an attack on your left front side.

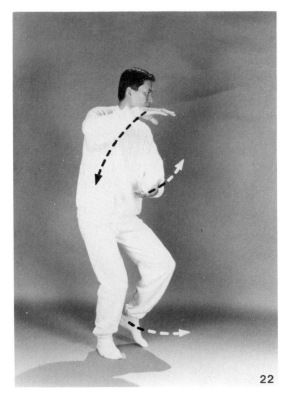

22

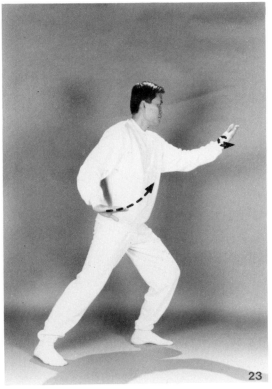

23

(13) Grasp the Bird's Tail, Left
Zuo Lan Jiao Wei

Movement 1: Turn your torso slightly left while extending your left hand forward with the palm turned down. Bring the right hand upward, with palm turning up, until it is below the left forearm. (See photo 24.) Now turn your torso to the right while pulling both hands down so that you draw an arc before the right side of the abdomen, finishing with your right hand extended sideways at shoulder level, palm up, and your left forearm lying across the chest, palm turned inward. At the same time, shift your weight to the right leg. (See photo 25.)

Eyes: Watch your left hand.

Breathing: Inhale.

Mind: Concentrate on the dantian.

Self-defense: Use both arms, hands, and palms to grasp an opponent's hand and pull it to your right side.

continued next page

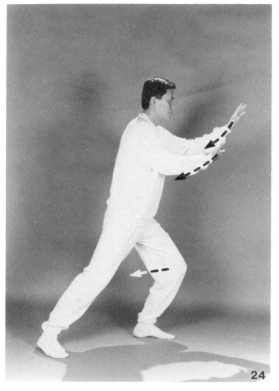

24

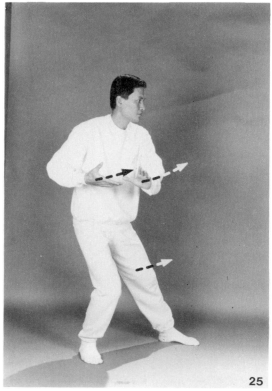

25

Movement 2: Turn your torso slightly left. Bend your right arm and place your right hand inside your left wrist. Turn your torso a little further left, and press both hands slowly forward, with the right palm facing forward, the left palm turned inward, and the left arm rounded. Meanwhile, shift your weight slowly to the left leg to form a bow step. (See photo 26.)

Eyes: Follow both hands.

Breathing: Exhale.

Mind: Visualize energy coming from the dantian through both arms to both hands.

Self-defense: Use both hands and palms to hit your opponent's chest in front of you.

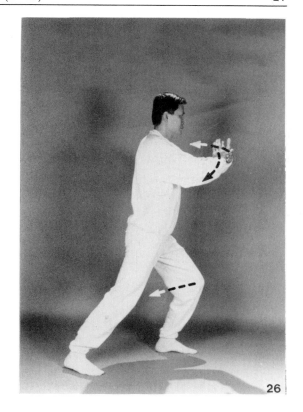

26

(14) Push, Left
Zuo An

Movement 1: Turn both palms downward as the right hand passes over the left wrist and moves forward and then right, ending level with the left hand. Separate hands a shoulder's width apart, and sit back as you shift your weight to the slightly bent right leg. Draw both hands back to the front of the abdomen, palms facing slightly downward to the front. (See photo 27.)

Eyes: Look forward.

Breathing: Inhale.

Mind: Concentrate on dantian.

Self-defense: Use both arms, hands, and palms to grasp your opponent's shoulders toward you and pull down.

Movement 2: Slowly transfer your weight to the left leg while pushing your hands forward and obliquely up, with palms facing forward, until your wrists are shoulder high. At the same time, bend the left knee into a bow step. (See photo 28.)

Eyes: Follow both hands.

Breathing: Exhale.

Mind: Visualize energy coming from the dantian through both arms to both hands.

Self-defense: Use both hands and palms to push your opponent's chest away.

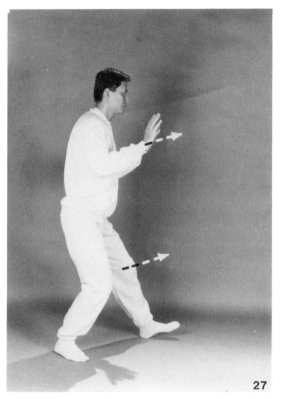

27

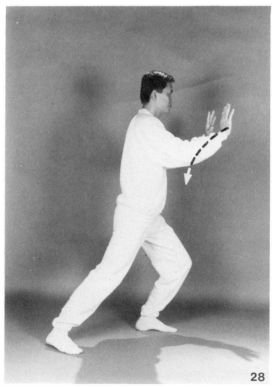

28

(15) Cross Hands
Shi Zi Shou

Movement: Shift your weight to the right leg, and turn your body to the right with your left heel touching the ground. Bend your right knee and sit back. Following the turn of the body, move both hands to your sides in a circular movement at shoulder level, with palms facing forward and elbows slightly bent. (See photo 29.) Slowly shift weight to the left leg, and turn the toes of your right foot inward. Then bring your right foot toward the left so that both feet are parallel and a shoulder's width apart. Gradually straighten the legs. At the same time, move both hands down and cross in front of your abdomen. Raise crossed hands to chest level with your wrists at shoulder level, your right hand on the outside, and your palms facing inward. (See photo 30.)

Eyes: Look forward.

Breathing: Inhale.

Mind: Concentrate on the dantian.

Self-defense: Use both arms and hands to protect your chest.

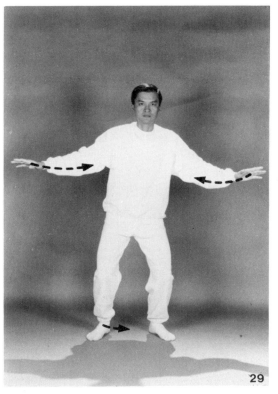

29

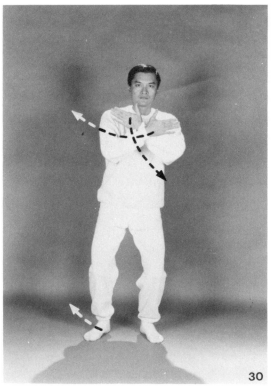

30

Second Sequence (16–30)

(16) Strike Right Fist
You Zai Chui

Movement: Turn your body to the right, move a step to your right side, and shift all your weight to the right foot, tracing your right fist and right arm counterclockwise in a circle 180 degrees, until your right elbow hangs at chin level and your right fist is above your head. Keep your left fist beside your left hip. (See photo 31.)

Eyes: Follow your right hand.

Breathing: Exhale.

Mind: Direct energy from the dantian to your right arm and fist.

Self-defense: Use your right fist and arm to protect yourself, especially your head, against an opponent's attack from your right side. At the same time, use your left fist and arm to block your left side in case an opponent tries to kick you there.

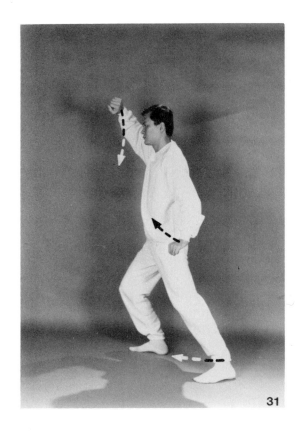

31

(17) Parting the Wild Horse's Mane, Left
Zuo Yei Ma Fen Zong

Movement 1: Shift your weight to the left and turn your torso slightly left; then, shift your weight slowly back to your right leg. Bring your right hand sideways up to shoulder level, with your palm facing downward, while your left palm is turned upward. Make a ball-holding gesture in front of the right side of your chest, with your right hand on top. (See photo 32.)

Eyes: Watch your right hand.

Breathing: Inhale.

Mind: Concentrate on the dantian.

Self-defense: Put more chi on both hands and palms.

Movement 2: Step forward and left with your left foot. Turn your torso a bit further left, and bend the left leg to form a bow step with the right leg naturally straightened. Shift your weight slowly to the left leg. Meanwhile, push out your rounded left forearm at shoulder level with the palm facing inward. Drop the right hand slowly to the side of your right hip, with the palm facing downward and fingers pointing forward. (See photo 33.)

Eyes: Follow the left hand.

Breathing: Exhale.

Mind: Visualize energy coming from the dantian through the left arm to the left hand.

Self-defense: Use your left arm, hand, and palm to protect yourself from attack from your left front side.

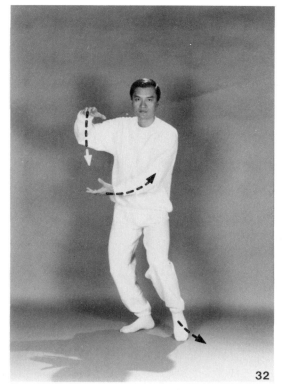

32

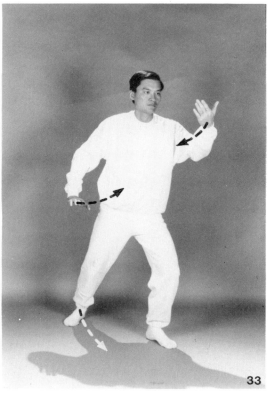

33

(18) Fist Under Elbow, Right
You Zhou Di Chui

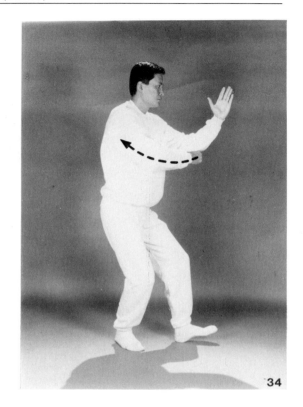

34

Movement: Move your right foot a step, bringing it close to your left foot. Shift your weight back to your right leg with your left heel touching the ground. Then turn your upper torso further to the left while extending your left arm in front of your chest. Hold your right fist and move it under the left elbow. (See photo 34.)

Eyes: Follow your left hand.

Breathing: Inhale first, then exhale.

Mind: Concentrate on the dantian first, then visualize energy coming from the dantian through both arms to the left hand and the right fist.

Self-defense: Use both arms, the left hand, and the right fist to protect yourself from attack in front of you.

(19) Drive the Monkey Away, Right
You Dao Ling Hou

Movement 1: Turn your body right, and open up your palm. Circle your right hand counterclockwise, downward, backwards, and upward, and extend it toward the back at shoulder height. At the same time, turn your left hand palm up, and extend it to the front at shoulder height. (See photo 35.)

Eyes: Follow your right hand.

Breathing: Inhale.

Mind: Concentrate on the dantian.

Self-defense: Use your left hand and arm to protect yourself from the left and front side, and use your right hand and arm to protect yourself from the right and back side.

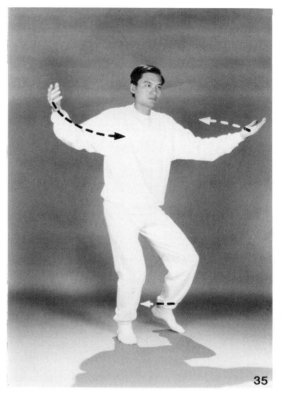

35

Movement 2: Turn your body left, and continue to make a circle with your right hand by bringing it forward and placing it beside your right ear with the palm forward and slightly downward. Then turn your left palm upward, draw it back and downward, and put it beside your left thigh. Draw your right hand downward, with your elbow bent, in front of your chest, with your fingers pointing slightly upward. At the same time, step back with your left foot with toes pointing directly in front, and shift your weight to it, curving your toes slightly inward. When most of your weight has been gradually shifted to your left foot, push your right hand forward with the elbow slightly bent and palm outward. (See photo 36.)

Eyes: Follow your right hand.

Breathing: Exhale.

Mind: Visualize energy coming from the dantian through your right arm to your right hand and right palm.

Self-defense: Use your right hand and palm to attack an opponent in front of you.

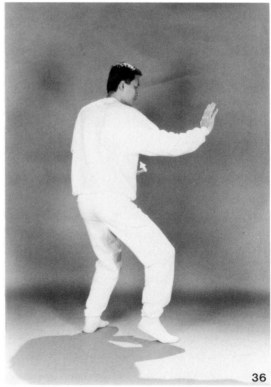

36

(20) Drive the Monkey Away, Left
Zuo Dao Ling Hou

Movement 1: Turn your body to the left and open your left palm up. Circle your left hand clockwise, downward, backwards, and upward, and extend it toward the back at shoulder height. At the same time, turn your right hand palm up, and extend it to the front at shoulder height. (See photo 37.)

Eyes: Follow your left hand.

Breathing: Inhale.

Mind: Concentrate on the dantian.

Self-defense: Use your right hand and arm to protect yourself from the right and front side, and use your left hand and arm to protect yourself from the left and back side.

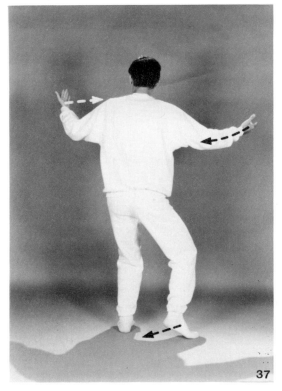

37

Movement 2: Turn your body to the right, and continue to circle with your left hand by bringing it forward and placing it beside your left ear with the palm forward and slightly downward. Then turn your right palm upward, draw it back and downward, and put it beside your right thigh. Draw the right hand downward, with the elbow bent, in front of your chest with fingers pointing slightly upward. At the same time, step back with your right foot with toes pointing directly in front, shift your weight to it, and curve your toes slightly inward. When you've shifted most of your weight gradually to your right foot, push your left hand forward with the elbow slightly bent and the palm outward. (See photo 38.)

Eyes: Follow your left hand.

Breathing: Exhale.

Mind: Visualize energy coming from the dantian through your left arm to your left hand and left palm.

Self-defense: Use your left hand and palm to attack an opponent in front of you.

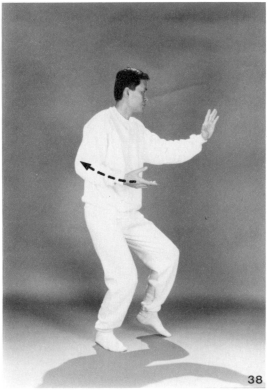

38

(21) Drive the Monkey Away, Right
You Dao Ling Hou

Movement 1: Turn your body to the right, open your palm up, and move your right hand in a counterclockwise circle, downward, backwards, and upward. Then extend it toward the back at shoulder height. At the same time, turn your left hand palm up, and extend it to the front at shoulder height. (See photo 39.)

Eyes: Follow your right hand.

Breathing: Inhale.

Mind: Concentrate on the dantian.

Self-defense: Use your left hand and arm to protect yourself from the left and front side, and use your right hand and arm to protect yourself from the right and back side.

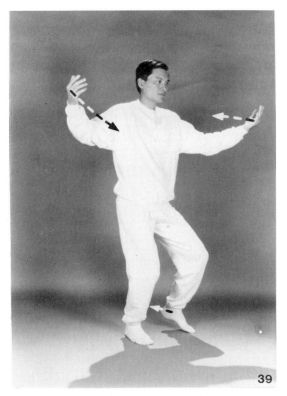

39

Movement 2: Turn your body left and continue to make your right hand circle by bringing it forward and placing it beside your right ear with the palm forward and slightly downward. Then turn your left palm upward, draw it back and downward, and put it beside your left thigh. Draw the right hand downward, with your elbow bent, in front of your chest with fingers pointing slightly upward. At the same time, step back with your left foot with toes pointing directly in front, shift your weight to it, and curve your toes slightly inward. When most of your weight has shifted gradually to your left foot, push your right hand forward with the elbow slightly bent and the palm outward. (See photo 40.)

Eyes: Follow your right hand.

Breathing: Exhale.

Mind: Visualize energy coming from the dantian through your right arm to your right hand and palm.

Self-defense: Use your right hand and palm to attack an opponent in front of you.

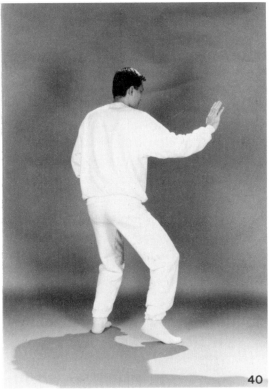

40

(22) Drive the Monkey Away, Left
Zuo Dao Ling Hou

Movement 1: Turn your body left, open your left palm up, and have your left hand circle clockwise, downward, backwards, and upward. Then extend it toward the back at shoulder height. At the same time, turn your right hand palm up, and extend it to the front at shoulder height. (See photo 41.)

Eyes: Follow your left hand.

Breathing: Inhale.

Mind: Concentrate on the dantian.

Self-defense: Use your right hand and arm to protect yourself from the right and front side, and use your left hand and arm to protect yourself from the left and back side.

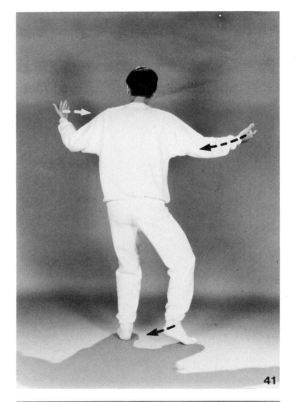

Movement 2: Turn your body to the right, and continue to make a circle with your left hand by bringing it forward and placing it, with the palm forward and slightly downward, beside your left ear. Then turn your right palm upward, draw it back and downward, and put it beside your right thigh. Draw your right hand downward, with the elbow bent, in front of your chest with your fingers pointing slightly upward. At the same time, step back with your right foot with toes pointing directly in front, shift your weight to it, and curve your toes slightly inward. When most of your weight has gradually shifted to your right foot, push your left hand forward with the elbow slightly bent and the palm outward. (See photo 42.)

Eyes: Follow your left hand.

Breathing: Exhale.

Mind: Visualize energy coming from the dantian through your left arm to your left hand and palm.

Self-defense: Use your left hand and palm to attack an opponent in front of you.

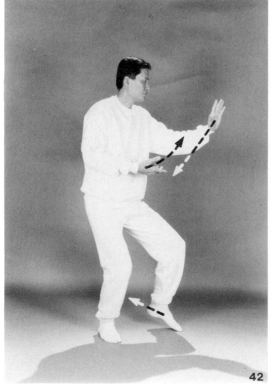

(23) Brush Left Knee and Push Out
Zuo Lou Xi Ao Bu

Movement: Turn the torso left 120 degrees, and take a big step forward with your left foot, with the heel touching the ground first. Brush your left knee with your left hand with palm downward, bringing it to rest beside the left thigh. Begin shifting your body weight to the left foot and curve the right foot slightly inward, turning on the heel. (See photo 43.) When 70 percent of your body weight is on your left foot, use the intrinsic energy of your entire body to push your right hand forward, with the elbow slightly bent. Then move your right foot close to your left foot with the toe touching the ground. (See photo 44.)

Eyes: Follow your right hand.

Breathing: First inhale, then exhale.

Mind: Concentrate on the dantian first; then visualize energy coming from the dantian through your right arm and hand to the right palm.

Self-defense: Use your right hand and palm to attack an opponent in front of you.

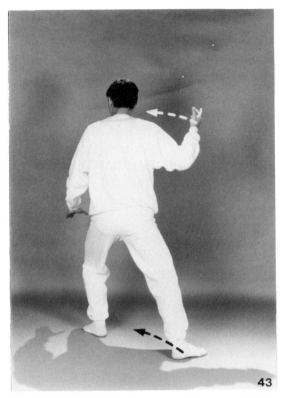

43

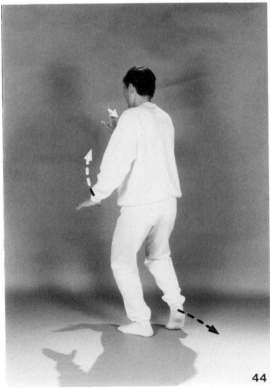

44

(24) Brush Right Knee and Push Out
You Lou Xi Ao Bu

Movement: Turn the torso to the right 180 degrees and take a big step forward with the right foot, heel touching the ground first. Brush the right knee with the right hand, palm downward, bringing it to rest beside the right thigh. Begin shifting your body weight to the right foot, and curve the left foot slightly inward, turning on the heel. (See photo 45.) When 70 percent of the body weight is on the right foot, with the intrinsic energy of your entire body, push the left hand forward, with the elbow slightly bent. Then move your left foot close to your right foot with the toe touching the ground. (See photo 46.)

Eyes: Follow your left hand.

Breathing: First inhale, then exhale.

Mind: Concentrate on the dantian first; then visualize energy coming from the dantian through the left arm and hand to the left palm.

Self-defense: Use your left hand and palm to attack an opponent in front of you.

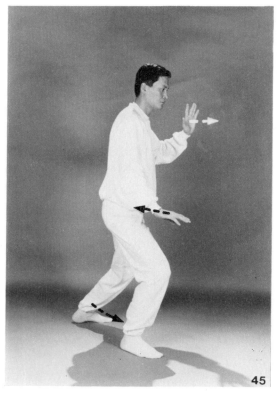

45

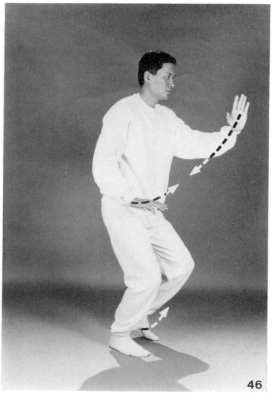

46

(25) Brush Left Knee and Push Out
Zuo Lou Xi Ao Bu

Movement: Turn your torso left 90 degrees, and take a big step forward with your left foot with your toe touching the ground first. Brush the left knee with the left hand, palm downward, bringing it to rest beside the left thigh. Begin shifting your body weight to the left foot and curve your right foot slightly inward, turning on the heel. (See photo 47.) When 70 percent of your body weight is on the left foot, use the intrinsic energy of your entire body to push the right hand forward, with your elbow slightly bent. Then move the right foot close to the left foot with the toe touching the ground. (See photo 48.)

Eyes: Follow your right hand.

Breathing: First inhale, then exhale.

Mind: Concentrate on the dantian first; then visualize energy coming from the dantian through the right arm and hand to your right palm.

Self-defense: Use your right hand and palm to attack an opponent in front of you.

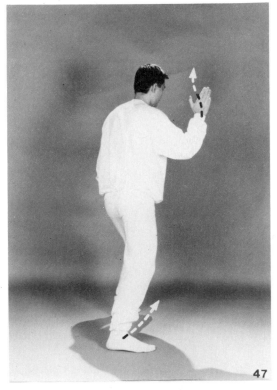

47

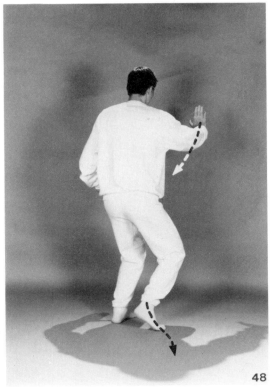

48

(26) Brush Right Knee and Push Out
You Lou Xi Ao Bu

Movement: Turn your torso to the right 180 degrees, and take a big step forward with your right foot, the heel touching the ground first. Brush the right knee with your right hand, palm downward, bringing it to rest beside your right thigh. Begin shifting your body weight to the right foot, and curve your left foot slightly inward, turning on the heel. (See photo 49.) When 70 percent of your body weight is on the right foot, with the intrinsic energy of your entire body, push your left hand forward, with the elbow slightly bent, then move your left foot close to your right foot with the toe touching the ground. (See photo 50.)

Eyes: Follow your left hand.

Breathing: First inhale, then exhale.

Mind: Concentrate on the dantian first; then visualize energy coming from the dantian through the left arm and hand to the left palm.

Self-defense: Use your left hand and palm to attack an opponent in front of you.

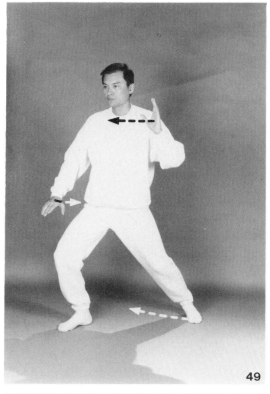

49

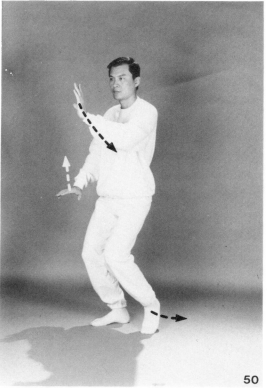

50

(27) Playing the Guitar and Push Out, Right
You Shou Hui Pi Pa

Movement 1: Move your left foot back a small step, shift your weight slightly left, and your right foot should touch the ground with the heel only, in line with the left heel. At the same time, bring your left hand along in a backward arc, palm facing right, to a position opposite the right elbow, raising the right hand with its palm facing left so that the fingers align with the mouth. The elbow should be slightly bent and the fingers point forward. This position simulates playing a guitar. (See photo 51.)

Eyes: Follow your right hand.

Breathing: Inhale.

Mind: Concentrate on your dantian.

Self-defense: Use both hands and palms to protect the upper half of your body from a frontal attack.

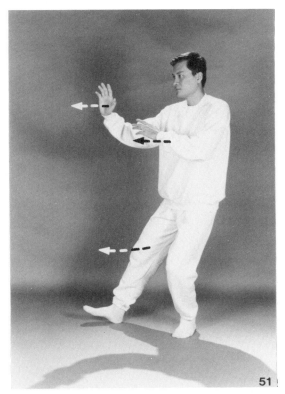

51

Movement 2: Extend your right foot forward a step; shift weight to the right leg. Turn the torso slightly to the right. Bend your left arm and place your left hand inside your right wrist. Turn the torso a little further right, and push both hands slowly forward with the left palm facing forward, the right palm inward, and the right arm rounded. Then move your left foot close to the right foot with the toe touching the ground. (See photo 52.)

Eyes: Follow both hands.

Breathing: Exhale.

Mind: Visualize energy coming from the dantian through both arms to both hands.

Self-defense: Use both hands and palms to hit your opponent's chest in front of you.

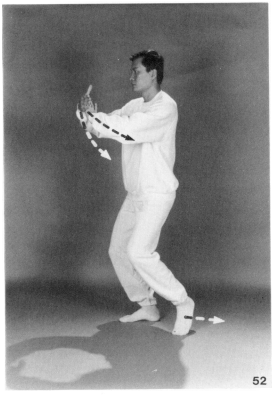

52

(28) Brush Right Knee and Punch Left Fist
You Lou Xi Ao Bu, Zuo Zai Chui

Movement 1: Move your left foot back a small step and shift your weight to your left foot. Move your right foot close to your left foot with your heel touching the ground. Have the right hand circle upward, backwards, and downward to the left side of the head. At the same time, circle the left hand clockwise, backwards, upward, and forward to the left ear. Then change the left palm slightly to a fist. (See photo 53.)

Eyes: Look forward.

Breathing: Inhale.

Mind: Concentrate on the dantian.

Self-defense: Use your right hand and arm and your left hand and arm to protect yourself from a frontal attack.

Movement 2: Turn your torso slightly to the right, and take a big step forward with your right foot, with the heel touching the ground first. Brush your right knee with your right hand, palm downward, bringing it to rest beside the right thigh. Begin shifting your body weight to the right foot, and curve the left foot slightly inward, turning on the heel. Punch your left fist down in front of your body. (See photo 54.)

Eyes: Follow your left hand.

Breathing: Exhale.

Mind: Visualize energy coming from the dantian through your left arm to your left fist.

Self-defense: Use your right hand and palm to protect your right knee from an opponent's kick, and use your left fist to attack an opponent in front of you.

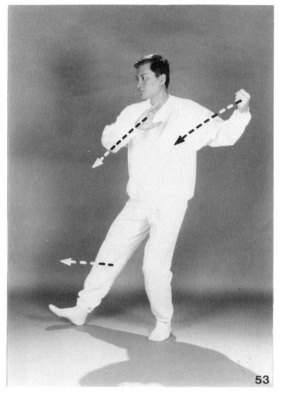

53

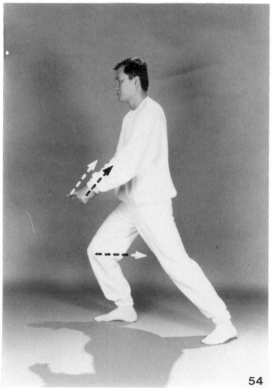

54

(29) Sit Down and Push Out Right Hand
You Bai She Tu Xing

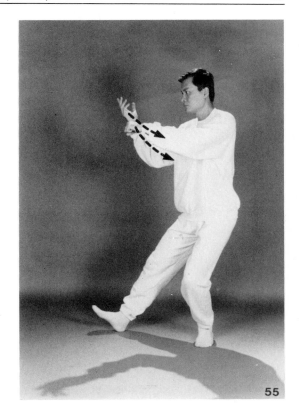

55

Movement 1: Shift your weight slightly to your left foot with the right heel touching the ground. At the same time, raise your right hand and left fist in front of your chest. Turn your torso left 90 degrees while turning the right heel; then shift your weight back to your right foot. Turn your torso to the left again 90 degrees. (See photo 55.)

Eyes: Follow your right hand.

Breathing: Inhale.

Mind: Concentrate on the dantian.

Self-defense: Use your right hand and left fist to protect yourself from a frontal attack.

continued next page

Movement 2: Take a big step forward with your left foot, heel touching the ground first. Change your left fist to an open palm and draw it back to beside your left hip. Begin shifting your body weight to the left foot, and curve the right foot slightly inward, turning on the heel. (See photo 56.) When 70 percent of your body weight is on the left foot, use the intrinsic energy of your entire body to push your right hand forward, elbow slightly bent. Bend your left knee, and close your right foot to your left foot to form a sitting posture. (See photo 57.)

Eyes: Follow your right hand.

Breathing: Exhale.

Mind: Visualize energy coming from the dantian through your right arm to your right hand and palm.

Self-defense: Use your left hand and palm to protect your left side from an opponent's attack, and use your right hand and palm to attack an opponent in front of you.

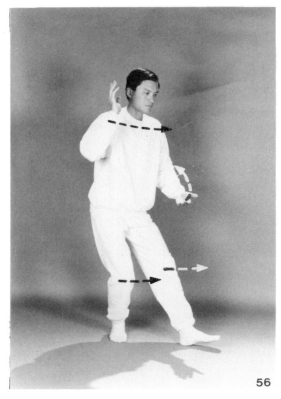

56

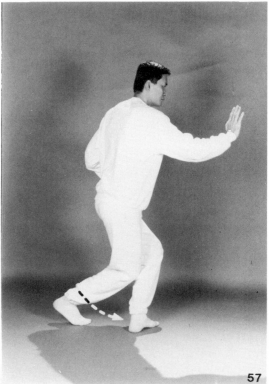

57

(30) Sit Down and Push Out Left Hand
Zuo Bai She Tu Xing

Movement: Take a big step forward with your right foot, heel touching the ground first. Draw your right hand back to beside your right hip. Begin shifting your body weight to the right foot, and curve the left foot slightly inward, turning on the heel. (See photo 58.) When 70 percent of your body weight is on the right foot, use the intrinsic energy of your entire body to push the left hand forward, elbow slightly bent. Bend your right knee and close your left foot to your right foot to form a sitting posture. (See photo 59.)

Eyes: Follow your left hand.

Breathing: Inhale first, then exhale.

Mind: Concentrate on the dantian first, then visualize energy coming from the dantian through your left arm to your left hand and palm.

Self-defense: Use your right hand and palm to protect your right side from an opponent's attack, and use your left hand and palm to attack an opponent in front of you.

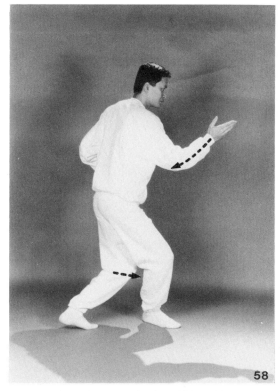

58

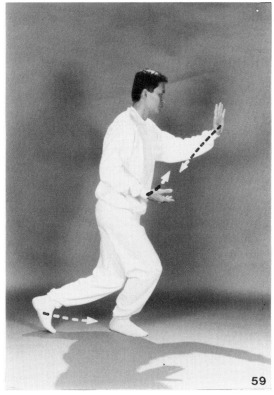

59

Third Sequence (31–45)

(31) Kick Right Heel
You Deng Jiao

Movement 1: Take a big step forward with your left foot, heel touching the ground first. Shift your weight slightly to your left foot. Draw your left hand back to beside the left hip while making a fist. Move your right hand counterclockwise—backwards and upward until it reaches the level of your right ear. (See photo 60.)

Eyes: Look forward.

Breathing: Inhale.

Mind: Concentrate on the dantian.

Self-defense: Use your left hand to protect your left side from an opponent's kick and your right hand to protect the right side of your head.

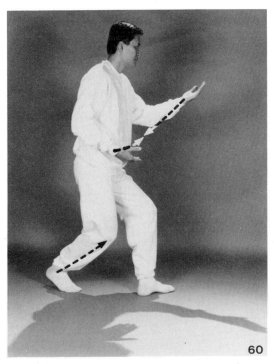

Movement 2: Bring your right foot beside your left foot and rest your toes on the floor. Extend your right hand to the right side of your body at shoulder height with your palm facing down. At the same time, raise your right leg, bent at the knee, and thrust the foot forward gradually until you touch your right hand. (See photo 61.)

Eyes: Follow your right hand.

Breathing: Exhale.

Mind: Visualize energy coming from the dantian through your right hip, thigh, and leg to your right foot.

Self-defense: Use your right leg and foot to attack an opponent in front of you.

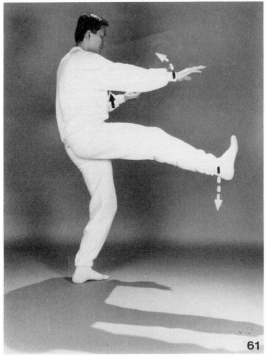

(32) Punch Right Fist
You Zai Chui

Movement: The right foot touches the floor; then shift your weight to the right foot slightly. Turn your torso left 90 degrees; then shift your weight to your left foot slightly. Move your left arm and hand clockwise to the left side of your face. Punch your right fist out from face level. (See photo 62.)

Eyes: Follow your right hand.

Breathing: Inhale first, then exhale.

Mind: Concentrate on the dantian first; then visualize energy coming from the dantian through your right arm to your right fist.

Self-defense: Use your left arm and hand to protect your head, and use your right fist to attack an opponent in front of you.

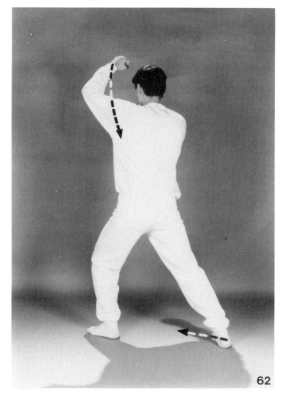

62

(33) Kick Left Heel
Zuo Deng Jiao

Movement 1: Shift your weight to the right foot, turn your torso left 90 degrees, and shift your weight back to the left foot. Take a big step forward with your right foot, heel touching the ground first. Shift your weight slightly to your right foot. Push out your right hand, and move your left hand back to the left side. (See photo 63.)

Eyes: Look forward.

Breathing: Inhale.

Mind: Concentrate on the dantian.

Self-defense: Use your right fist to protect your right side from an opponent's kick and your left hand to protect the left side of your head.

continued next page

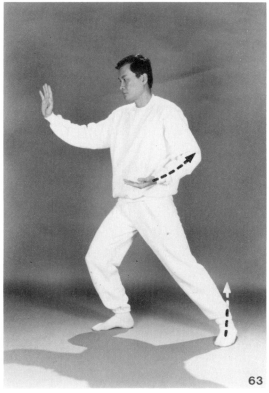

63

Movement 2: Bring your left foot to the side of your right foot and rest your toes on the floor. Extend your left hand to the left side of your body at shoulder height with palm facing down. At the same time, raise your left leg, bent at the knee, and thrust the foot gradually forward until you touch your left hand. (See photo 64.)

Eyes: Follow your left hand.

Breathing: Exhale.

Mind: Visualize energy coming from the dantian through your left hip, thigh, and leg to your left foot.

Self-defense: Use your left leg and foot to attack an opponent in front of you.

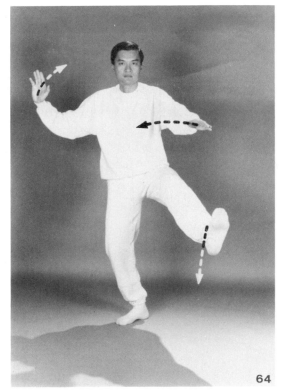

64

(34) Punch Left Fist
Zuo Zai Chui

Movement: Touch the floor with your left foot, shift your weight to the left foot slightly, and turn your torso left 90 degrees. Move your right arm and hand clockwise to the right side of your face, punch your left fist out at face level. (See photo 65.)

Eyes: Follow your left hand.

Breathing: Inhale first, then exhale.

Mind: Concentrate on the dantian first; then visualize energy coming from the dantian through your left arm to your left fist.

Self-defense: Use your right arm and hand to protect your head, and use your left fist to attack an opponent in front of you.

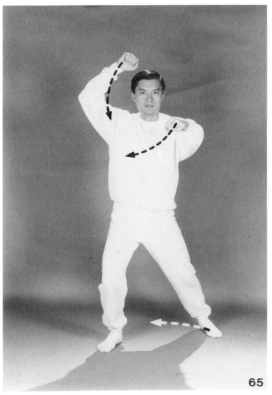

65

(35) Parting the Wild Horse's Mane, Left
Zuo Yei Ma Fen Zong

Movement 1: Turn your torso slightly to the right, and slowly shift your weight to the right leg. At the same time, bring your right hand sideways up to shoulder height, with palm facing downward, while your left palm is turned upward. Make a ball-holding gesture in front of the right side of your chest, with the right hand on top. (See photo 66.)

Eyes: Watch right hand.

Breathing: Inhale.

Mind: Concentrate on the dantian.

Self-defense: Put more chi on both hands and palms.

Movement 2: Turn your torso left 120 degrees and take a step forward with your left foot. Turn your torso a bit further left and bend your left leg to form a bow step with the right leg naturally straightened. Shift your weight slowly to the left leg. Meanwhile, push out your rounded left forearm at shoulder level while forming a fist. Put the right hand on the wrist of the left hand with the right palm facing outside. (See photo 67.)

Eyes: Follow both hands.

Breathing: Exhale.

Mind: Visualize energy coming from the dantian through both arms to both hands.

Self-defense: Use both arms, hands, fists, and palms to protect yourself from attack from the front. Also attack the opponent in front of you.

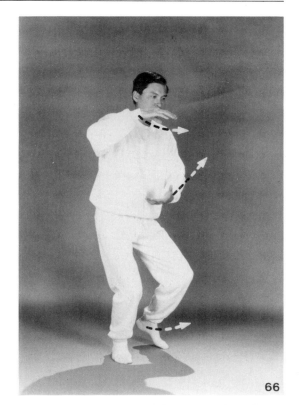

66

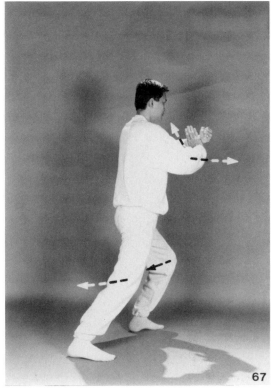

67

(36) Hands Circle and Press Down
Xia Shi

Movement 1: Both hands circle upward, outward, then downward, and inward, with the right hand clockwise and the left hand counterclockwise, finishing with the left fist under the right elbow. At the same time, move your right foot close to your left foot with the toe touching the ground. (See photos 68 and 69.)

Eyes: Follow both hands.

Breathing: Inhale.

Mind: Concentrate on the dantian.

Self-defense: Use both arms and hands to protect yourself from attack in front of you.

continued next page

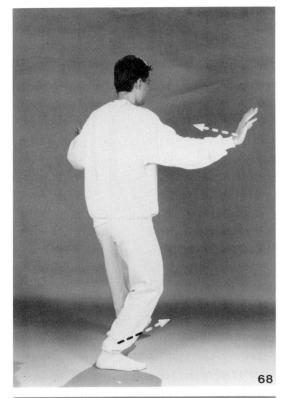

68

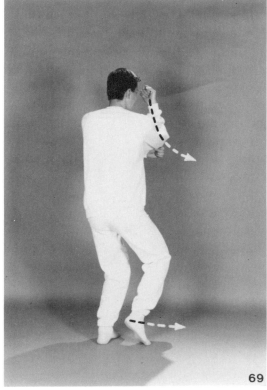

69

Movement 2: Slowly crouch on the left leg, stretching the right leg sideways towards it. Extend the right hand sideways along the inner side of the right leg, with the palm facing forward. Draw the left hand clockwise around the left side of your body, finishing beside your left hip while forming a fist. Using your heel as a pivot, turn the toes of your right foot slightly outward so that they align with your outstretched leg. Turn toes of the left foot inward. Turn your torso slightly to the right, and then raise it slowly, moving forward. (See photo 70.)

Eyes: Follow your right hand.

Breathing: Exhale.

Mind: Visualize energy coming from the dantian through your right arm to your right hand.

Self-defense: Use your left hand and fist to protect the left side of your body, and use your right hand and palm to attack an opponent in front of you.

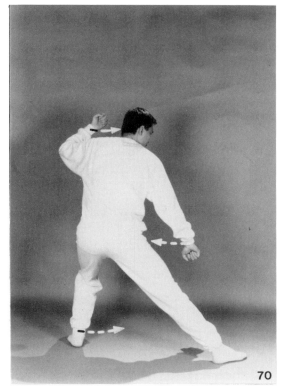

(37) Stand on One Leg, Left and Right
Zuo You Jing Ji Du Li

Movement 1: Raise the left foot gradually and bend your left knee so that your thigh is level. At the same time, open your left hand and swing your arm past the outer side of your left leg, then upward to the front, until your bent elbow is just above the left knee, with fingers pointing up and the palm facing the right side. Lower your right hand to beside your right hip with palm facing downward. (See photo 71.)

Eyes: Follow your left hand.

Breathing: Inhale.

Mind: Concentrate on the dantian first; then visualize energy coming from the dantian

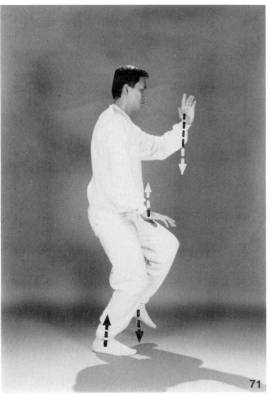

continued next page

through your left arm to your left hand and through your left thigh to your left knee and leg.

Self-defense: Use your right hand and palm to protect the right side of your body. Use your left hand to attack an opponent's jaw, and use your left leg and knee to attack the lower part of an opponent's body.

Movement 2: Move your left foot down, touching the ground, and shift your weight to your left foot. Raise your right foot gradually and bend your right knee until your thigh is level. At the same time, swing your right hand past the outer side of your right leg and then upward to the front, until the bent elbow is just above your right knee, with fingers pointing up and your palm facing the left side. Lower your left hand so that it's beside your left hip, with the palm facing downward. (See photo 72.)

Eyes: Follow your right hand.

Breathing: Exhale.

Mind: Concentrate on the dantian first; then visualize energy coming from the dantian through your right arm to your right hand and through your right thigh to your right knee and leg.

Self-defense: Use your left hand and palm to protect the left side of your body, and use your right hand to attack an opponent's jaw. Use your right leg and knee to attack the lower part of an opponent's body.

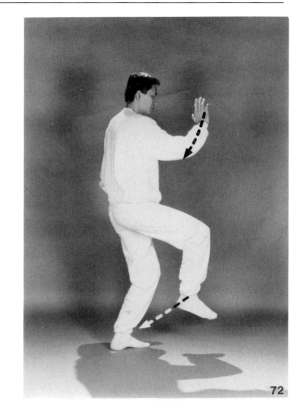

72

(38) Grasp the Bird's Tail, Left
Zuo Lan Jiao Wei

Movement 1: Move your right foot down, touching the ground. Turn your torso slightly left while extending your left hand forward with the palm turned down. Bring your right hand upward, with the palm turning up, until it is below your left forearm. (See photo 73.) Then turn your torso to the right while pulling both hands down so that you draw an arc before the right side of your abdomen. Finish with your right hand extended sideways at shoulder level, palm up, and with your left forearm lying across your chest, palm turned inward. At the same time, shift your weight to the right leg. (See photo 74.)

Eyes: Watch the left hand.

Breathing: Inhale

Mind: Concentrate on the dantian.

Self-defense: Use both arms, hands, and palms to grasp an opponent's hand and pull it to your right side.

continued next page

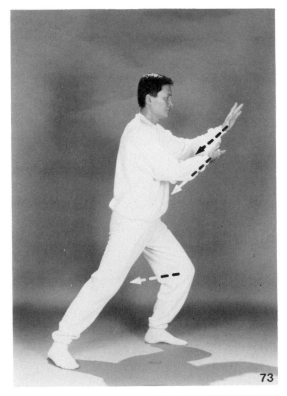

73

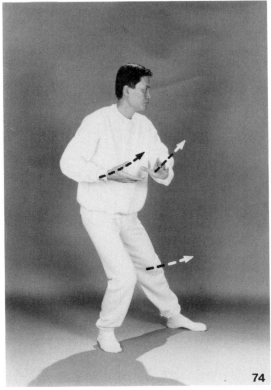

74

Movement 2: Turn the torso slightly to the left. Bend your right arm and place your right hand inside your left wrist. Turn your torso a little farther left, and press both hands slowly forward, with the right palm facing forward, the left palm turned inward, and the left arm rounded. Meanwhile, shift your weight slowly to the left leg to form a bow step. (See photo 75.)

Eyes: Follow both hands.

Breathing: Exhale.

Mind: Visualize energy coming from the dantian through both arms to both hands.

Self-defense: Use both hands and palms to hit your opponent's chest in front of you.

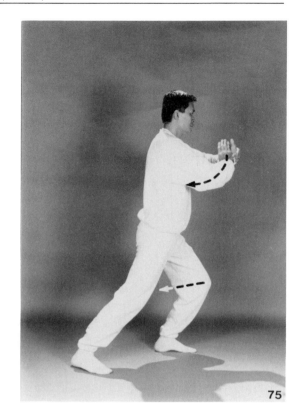

75

(39) Push Hands, Left
Zuo An

Movement 1: Turn both palms downward as your right hand passes over your left wrist and moves forward and then right, ending level with your left hand. Separate hands a shoulder's width apart, and sit back as you shift your weight to the slightly bent right leg. Draw both hands back to the front of your abdomen, with palms facing slightly downward to the front. (See photo 76.)

Eyes: Look forward.

Breathing: Inhale.

Mind: Concentrate on the dantian.

Self-defense: Use both arms, hands, and palms to grasp your opponent's shoulders, pulling them toward you and down.

Movement 2: Slowly transfer your weight to the left leg while pushing your hands forward and obliquely up, with palms facing forward, until your wrists are shoulder high. At the same time, bend your left knee into a bow step. (See photo 77.)

Eyes: Follow both hands.

Breathing: Exhale.

Mind: Visualize energy coming from the dantian through both arms to both hands.

Self-defense: Use both hands and palms to push your opponent's chest away.

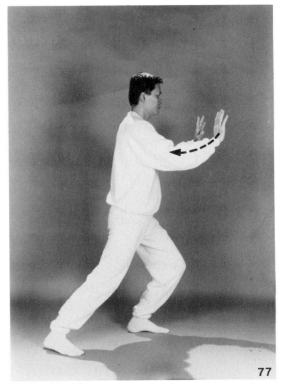

77

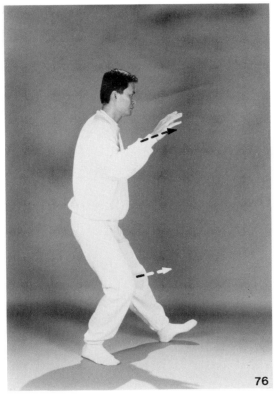

76

(40) First Waving Hands in the Cloud
Yi Yun Shou

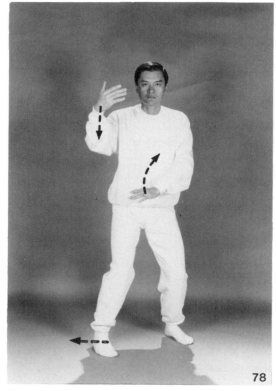

78

Movement 1: Move your right hand down to the side of your left hip. Turn your torso to the right, and lower your left hand near your abdomen with the palm inward. Raise your right hand to neck height with the palm facing you. Turn your torso gradually to the right and shift your weight to the right foot. Continue to turn your torso together with both hands to the right. Shift all your weight to the right foot until your left hand, palm up, is near the abdomen and your right hand, palm down, is near the neck. Assume a ball-holding stance. Move your left foot a step closer to your right foot. (See photo 78.)

Eyes: Follow your right hand and palm.

Breathing: Inhale.

Mind: Concentrate on the dantian first; then visualize energy coming from the dantian through both arms to both hands and palms.

Self-defense: Protect yourself from an attack in front.

Movement 2: Turn your torso left, and lower your right hand near your abdomen with palm inward. Raise your left hand to neck height with the palm facing you. Turn your torso gradually left and shift your weight to the left foot. Continue to turn your torso with both hands left. Shift your weight to your left foot until your right hand, palm up, is near your abdomen and your left hand, palm down, is near your neck. Assume a ball-holding stance. (See photo 79.)

Eyes: Follow your left hand and palm.

Breathing: Exhale.

Mind: Concentrate on the dantian first; then visualize energy coming from the dantian through both arms to both hands and palms.

Self-defense: Protect yourself from an attack in front.

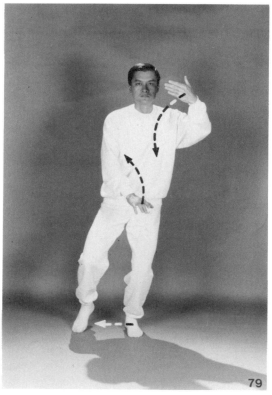

79

(41) Second Waving Hands in the Cloud
Er Yun Shou

Movement 1: Move your right foot a step to the right. Turn your torso to the right, and lower your left hand to your abdomen with palm inward. Raise your right hand to neck height with the palm facing you. Turn your torso gradually right and shift your weight to the right foot. Continue to turn your torso with both hands right. Shift your weight to your right foot until your left hand, palm up, is near your abdomen and your right hand, palm down, is near your neck. Assume a ball-holding stance. Move your left foot a step, moving it close to your right foot. (See photo 80.)

Eyes: Follow your right hand and palm.

Breathing: Inhale.

Mind: Concentrate on the dantian first; then visualize energy coming from the dantian through both arms to both hands and palms.

Self-defense: Protect yourself from attack in front of you.

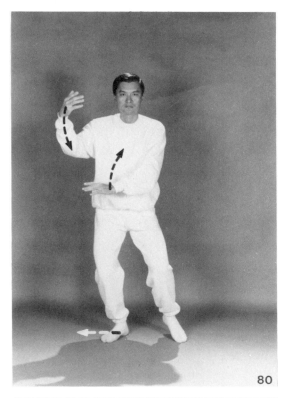

Movement 2: Turn your torso left, and lower your right hand near your abdomen with palm inward. Raise your left hand to neck height with your palm facing you. Turn your torso gradually left and shift your weight to your left foot. Continue to turn your torso with both hands left. Shift your weight to the left foot until your right hand, palm up, is near your abdomen and the left hand, palm down, is near your neck. Assume a ball-holding stance. (See photo 81.)

Eyes: Follow your left hand and palm.

Breathing: Exhale.

Mind: Concentrate on the dantian first; then visualize energy coming from the dantian through both arms to both hands and palms.

Self-defense: Protect yourself from attack in front of you.

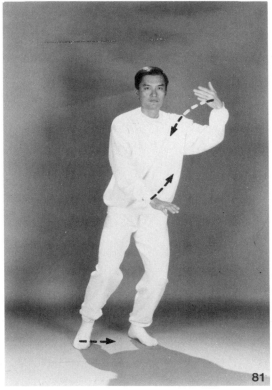

(42) Parting the Wild Horse's Mane, Right
You Yei Ma Fen Zong

Movement 1: Shift your weight to the left foot, and turn your torso slightly to the left. Move your right foot close to the left foot with the big toe touching the ground. At the same time, bring your left hand sideways, up to shoulder level, palm facing downward, while your right hand moves back near your left hip with palm facing upward. Assume a ball-holding stance to the left of your chest, with left hand on top. (See photo 82.)

Eyes: Follow your left hand.

Breathing: Inhale.

Mind: Concentrate on the dantian.

Self-defense: Use both hands to protect your left front chest.

Movement 2: Take a step forward with your right foot. Turn your torso a bit further right and bend your right leg to form a bow step with your left leg naturally straightened. Shift your weight slowly to the right leg. Meanwhile, push out the rounded right forearm at shoulder level with your palm facing inward. Drop your left hand slowly to the side of your left hip, palm facing downward and fingers pointing forward. (See photo 83.)

Eyes: Follow the right hand.

Breathing: Exhale.

Mind: Visualize energy coming from the dantian through your right arm to your right hand and palm.

Self-defense: Use your right arm, hand, and palm to protect yourself from attack on your right front side.

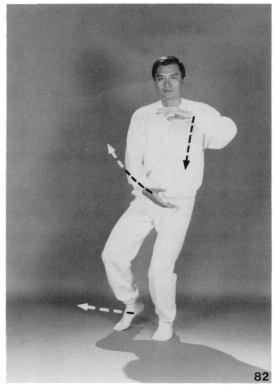

82

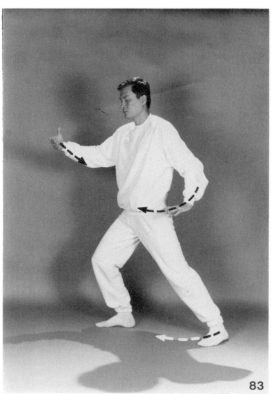

83

(43) Parting the Wild Horse's Mane, Left
Zuo Yei Ma Fen Zong

Movement 1: Turn your torso slightly to the right, move your left foot close to your right foot with the big toe touching the ground. At the same time, bring your right hand sideways up to shoulder height, palm facing downward, while your left hand moves back near your right hip with the palm facing upward. Assume a ball-holding gesture on the right side of your chest, with right hand on top. (See photo 84.)

Eyes: Follow your right hand.

Breathing: Inhale.

Mind: Concentrate on the dantian.

Self-defense: Use both hands to protect your right front chest.

Movement 2: Take a step forward with your left foot. Turn your torso a bit farther left and bend your left leg to form a bow step with the right leg naturally straightened. Shift your weight slowly to your left leg. Meanwhile, push out the rounded left forearm at shoulder level with palm facing forward. Drop your right hand slowly to the side of your right hip while making a fist. (See photo 85.)

Eyes: Follow the left hand.

Breathing: Exhale.

Mind: Visualize energy coming from the dantian through your left arm to your left hand and palm.

Self-defense: Use your left arm, hand, and palm to protect yourself from attack from your left front side.

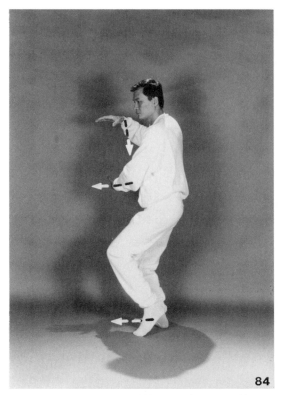

84

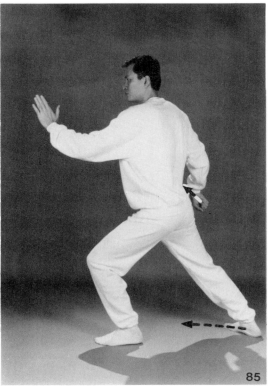

85

(44) Kick with Right Heel
You Deng Jiao

Movement 1: Both hands circle downward and then inward and upward until they cross in front of your chest. Turn both palms inward, with the back of your left hand against the inside of your right wrist. At the same time, bring your right foot beside your left foot and rest your toes on the floor. (See photo 86.)

Eyes: Look forward.

Breathing: Inhale.

Mind: Concentrate on the dantian.

Self-defense: Use both hands and palms to protect your chest from attack in front of you.

Movement 2: Separate hands, extending them sideways at shoulder level, with elbows slightly bent and palms turned outward. At the same time, raise your right leg, bent at the knee, and thrust the foot gradually forward. (See photo 87.)

Eyes: Follow your right hand.

Breathing: Exhale.

Mind: Visualize energy coming from the dantian through your right arm to your right hand and palm, as well as through your right leg to your right foot.

Self-defense: Use your right hand and right foot to attack an opponent in front on your right side.

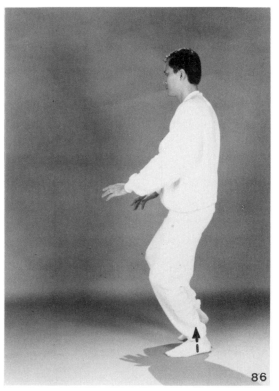

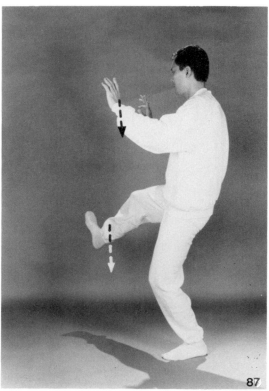

(45) Kick with Left Heel
Zuo Deng Jiao

Movement 1: Put your right foot down, touching the ground, and shift your weight slightly to your right foot. At the same time, have both hands circle downward, then inward and upward until they cross in front of your chest, with both palms turned inward and with the back of your right hand against the inside of your left wrist. At the same time, bring your left foot beside your right, and rest your toes on the floor. (See photo 88.)

Eyes: Look forward.

Breathing: Inhale.

Mind: Concentrate on the dantian.

Self-defense: Use both hands and palms to protect your chest from attack in front of you.

Movement 2: Separate hands, extending them sideways at shoulder level, with elbows slightly bent and palms turned outward. At the same time, raise your left leg, bent at the knee, and thrust the foot gradually forward. (See photo 89.)

Eyes: Follow your left hand.

Breathing: Exhale.

Mind: Visualize energy coming from the dantian through your left arm to your left hand and palm, as well as through your left leg to your left foot.

Self-defense: Use your left hand and left foot to attack an opponent in front on your left side.

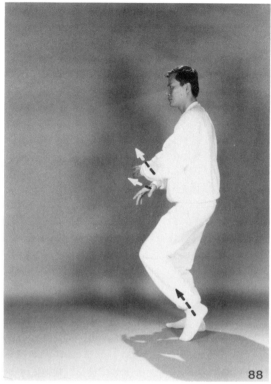

88

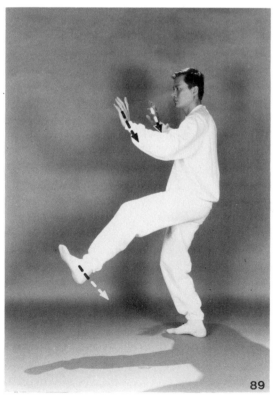

89

Fourth Sequence (46–60)

(46) Brush Left Knee and Punch Down
Zuo Lou Xi Ao Bu, You Zai Chui

Movement 1: Put your left foot down with the heel touching the ground. Have both hands circle downward and inward until they touch each other with the left fist on top of the right palm in front of the abdomen. (See photo 90.)

Eyes: Look forward.

Breathing: Inhale.

Mind: Concentrate on the dantian.

Self-defense: Use both hands to protect your chest and abdomen.

Movement 2: Move your left foot a big step forward with the heel touching the ground first. Shift your weight slightly to your left foot. At the same time, brush your left knee with the left hand, palm backward, bringing it to rest beside your left thigh. When 70 percent of your body weight is on the left foot, use the intrinsic energy of your entire body to punch the right fist forward and downward, with the elbow slightly bent. (See photo 91.)

Eyes: Follow your right hand and fist.

Breathing: Exhale.

Mind: Visualize energy coming from the dantian through your right arm to your right hand and fist.

Self-defense: Use your left hand and palm to protect your left knee from an opponent's kick, and use your right hand and fist to attack an opponent in front of you.

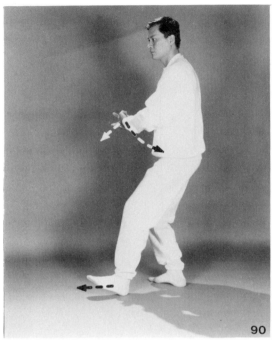

90

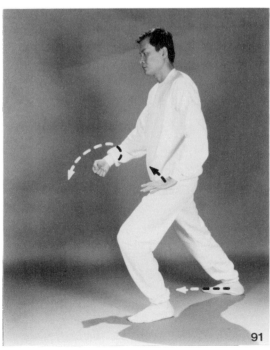

91

(47) Needle at the Bottom of the Sea
Hai Di Jen

Movement: Take half a step forward with your right foot. Shift your weight onto the right leg as your left foot moves forward with the toes coming down on the floor to form a left "empty" step. (See photo 92.) At the same time, turn your body slightly to the right, lower your right hand in front of your body, then raise it up beside your right ear, and thrust it obliquely downward in front of your body, with palm facing left and fingers

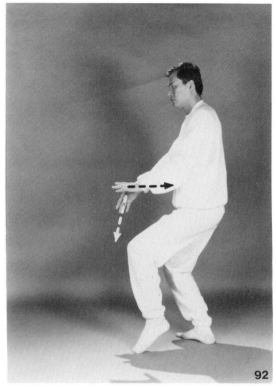

92

pointing obliquely downward. Simultaneously, make an arc forward and downward with your left hand to beside your left hip with the palm facing downward and fingers pointing forward. (See photo 93.)

Eyes: Follow your right hand.

Breathing: First inhale, then exhale.

Mind: Concentrate on the dantian first; then visualize energy coming from the dantian through your right arm to your right hand and palm.

Self-defense: Use your left hand and palm to protect your left side, and use your right hand and palm to attack an opponent in front of you.

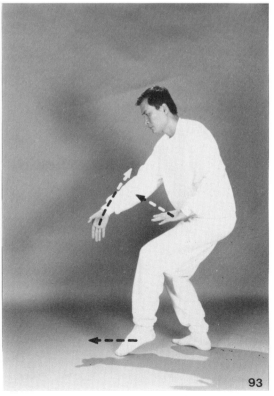

93

(48) Flash the Arm, Left
Zuo Shan Tong Bei

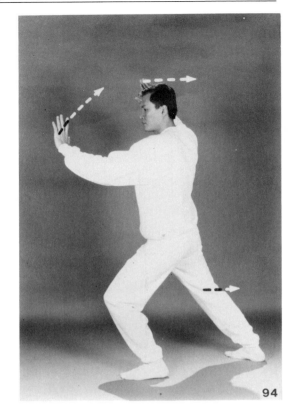

94

Movement: Turn the body slightly to the right. Step forward with your left foot to form a bow step. Shift your weight to your left foot. At the same time, raise your right arm with elbow bent until your hand stops just above your right temple. Turn the palm obliquely upward with the thumb pointing downward. Raise your left hand slightly, and push it forward at nose level with the palm facing forward. (See photo 94.)

Eye: Follow your left hand.

Breathing: First inhale, then exhale.

Mind: Concentrate on the dantian first; then visualize energy coming from the dantian through both arms to both hands and palms.

Self-defense: Use your right hand and palm to protect the right side of your head, and use your left hand and palm to attack an opponent in front of you.

(49) Turn Around and Kick with Right Heel
You Deng Jiao

Movement 1: Shift your weight to your right foot. Turn your torso right 120 degrees, with the toes of your left foot turned inward and the heel touching the ground. Then shift your weight back to your left foot. Circle both hands downward and then inward and upward until they cross in front of your chest, with both palms turned inward and the back of your left hand against the inside of your right wrist. At the same time, bring your right foot beside your left foot and rest your toes on the floor. (See photo 95.)

Eyes: Look forward.

Breathing: Inhale.

Mind: Concentrate on the dantian.

Self-defense: Use both hands and palms to protect your chest from an attack in front of you.

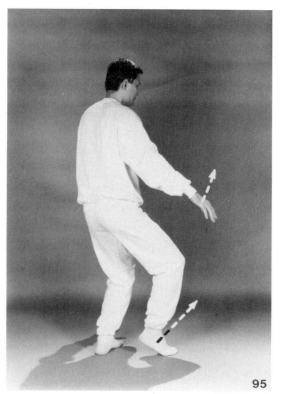
95

Movement 2: Separate your hands, extending them sideways at shoulder level, with elbows slightly bent and palms turned outward. At the same time, raise your right leg, bent at the knee, and thrust your foot gradually forward. (See photo 96.)

Eyes: Follow your right hand.

Breathing: Exhale.

Mind: Visualize energy coming from the dantian through your right arm to your right hand and palm, as well as through your right leg to your right foot.

Self-defense: Use your right hand and right foot to attack an opponent in front and to your right.

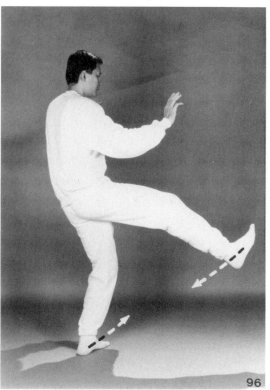
96

(50) Kick with Left Heel
Zuo Deng Jiao

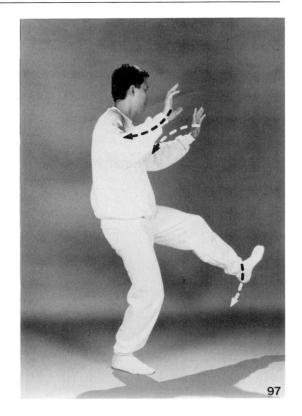

97

Movement 1: Put your right foot down, touching the ground, and shift your weight slightly to your right foot. At the same time, circle both hands downward and then inward and upward until they cross in front of your chest, with both palms turned inward and the back of your right hand against the inside of your left wrist. At the same time, bring your left foot beside your right, and rest your toes on the floor.

Eyes: Look forward.

Breathing: Inhale.

Mind: Concentrate on the dantian.

Self-defense: Use both hands and palms to protect your chest from an attack in front of you.

Movement 2: Separate hands, extending them sideways at shoulder level, with elbows slightly bent and palms turned outward. At the same time, raise your left leg, bent at the knee, and thrust your foot gradually forward. (See photo 97.)

Eyes: Follow your left hand.

Breathing: Exhale.

Mind: Visualize energy coming from the dantian through your left arm to your left hand and palm, as well as through your left leg to your left foot.

Self-defense: Use your left hand and left foot to attack an opponent in front and to your left.

(51) Brush Left Knee and Twist Step
Zuo Lou Xi Ao Bu

Movement 1: Put your left foot down with the heel touching the ground. Make the left hand circle clockwise, backward, and upward to the right ear. The palm should face outward and be slightly inclined downward with the elbow bent. (See photo 98.)

Eyes: Follow your left hand.

Breathing: Inhale.

Mind: Concentrate on the dantian.

Self-defense: Use your left hand to protect yourself from an attack in front of you.

Movement 2: Turn the torso slightly to the left and take a big step forward with the left foot, with the heel touching the ground first. Brush the left knee with the left hand, palm backward, bringing it to rest beside the left thigh. Begin shifting the body weight to the left foot and curve the right foot slightly inward, turning on the heel. When 70 percent of your body weight is on the left foot, use the intrinsic energy of your entire body to push the right hand forward, with the elbow slightly bent. (See photo 99.)

Eyes: Follow your right hand.

Breathing: Exhale.

Mind: Visualize energy coming from the dantian through your right arm to your right hand and palm.

Self-defense: Use your left hand and palm to protect your left knee from an opponent's kick, and use your right hand and palm to attack an opponent in front of you.

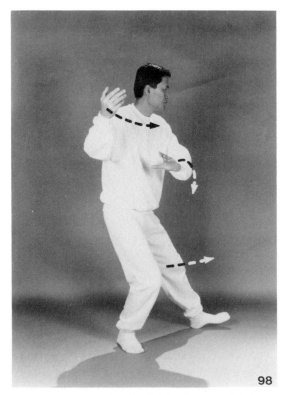

98

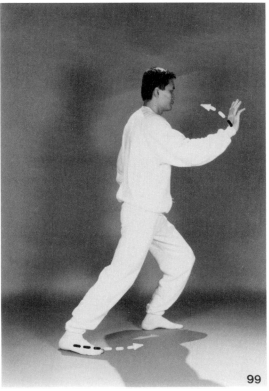

99

(52) Brush Right Knee and Twist Step
You Lou Xi Ao Bu

Movement 1: Move your right foot close to your left foot with the toe touching the ground. Have the right hand circle counterclockwise, backwards, and upward to the left ear. The palm should face outward and be slightly inclined downward with the elbow bent. Have the left hand circle clockwise, backwards, upward, and forward to the left side of your head. (See photo 100.)

Eyes: Follow your right hand.

Breathing: Inhale.

Mind: Concentrate on the dantian.

Self-defense: Use your right hand to protect yourself from an attack in front of you.

Movement 2: Turn your torso slightly to the right, and take a big step forward with the right foot, heel touching the ground first. Brush the right knee with the right hand, palm backwards, bringing it to rest beside the right thigh. Begin shifting your body weight to the right foot, and curve the left foot slightly inward, turning on your heel. When 70 percent of your body weight is on the right foot, use the intrinsic energy of your entire body to push the left hand forward, with the elbow slightly bent. (See photo 101.)

Eyes: Follow your left hand.

Breathing: Exhale.

Mind: Visualize energy coming from the dantian through your left arm to your left hand and palm.

Self-defense: Use your right hand and palm to protect your right knee from an opponent's kick, and use your left hand and palm to attack an opponent in front of you.

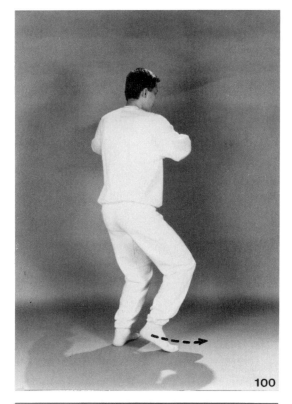

100

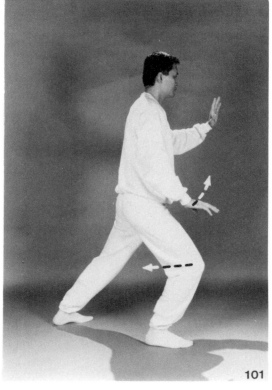

101

(53) Press Right Hand
You An

Movement 1: Shift your weight to your left foot, have your right hand circle counter-clockwise, upward, forward, inward, and backwards until touching your left palm with your right wrist in front of your chest. (See photo 102.)

Eyes: Follow your right hand.

Breathing: Inhale.

Mind: Concentrate on the dantian.

Self-defense: Use both hands to protect your chest from an attack in front of you.

Movement 2: Shift your weight to your right foot, bending the left knee slightly. Draw your left hand backwards, and extend your right hand forward until your left hand is near your abdomen with palm up and your right hand is in front, over your left hand with palm forward and elbow slightly bent. (See photo 103.)

Eyes: Follow your right hand.

Breathing: Exhale.

Mind: Visualize energy coming from the dantian through your right arm to your right hand and palm.

Self-defense: Use your right hand and palm to attack an opponent in front of you. At the same time, use the left hand to protect your left front side.

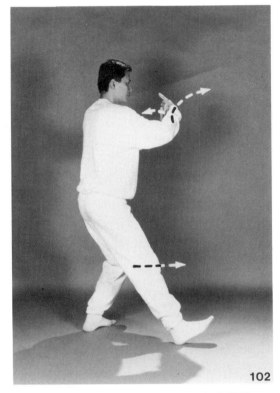

102

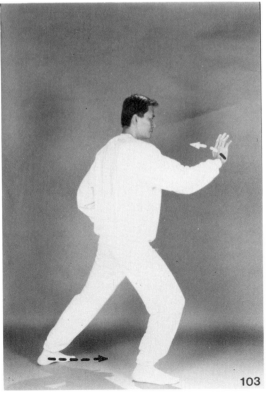

103

(54) Cross Fists
Shi Zi Chui

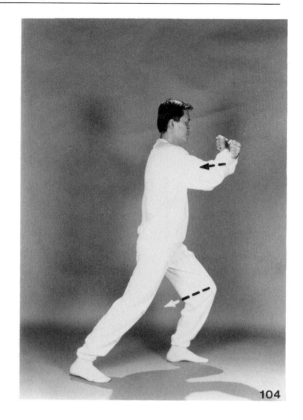

104

Movement: Move the left foot a step forward; then shift your weight slightly to the left foot. At the same time, have both hands circle downward, then inward and upward until they cross in front of your chest while making fists with the palm side turned inward and the back of your right hand against the inside of your left wrist. (See photo 104.)

Eyes: Follow both hands.

Breathing: First inhale, then exhale.

Mind: Concentrate on the dantian first; then visualize energy coming from the dantian through both arms to both fists.

Self-defense: Use both arms, hands, and fists to protect yourself and to attack an opponent in front of you.

(55) Push Hands, Left
Zuo An

Movement 1: Turn both palms downward as the right hand passes over the left wrist and moves forward and then right, ending level with the left hand. Separate hands a shoulder's width apart, and sit back as you shift your weight to the slightly bent right leg. Draw both hands back in front of the abdomen, palms facing slightly downward to the front. (See photo 105.)

Eyes: Look forward.

Breathing: Inhale.

Mind: Concentrate on the dantian.

Self-defense: Use both arms, hands, and palms to grasp your opponent's shoulders, pulling them toward you and down.

Movement 2: Slowly transfer your weight to your left leg while pushing your hands forward and obliquely up, with palms facing forward, until wrists are shoulder-high. At the same time, bend the left knee into a bow step. (See photo 106.)

Eyes: Follow both hands.

Breathing: Exhale.

Mind: Visualize energy coming from the dantian through both arms to both hands.

Self-defense: Use both hands and palms to push your opponent's chest away.

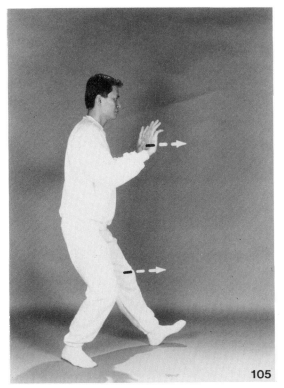

105

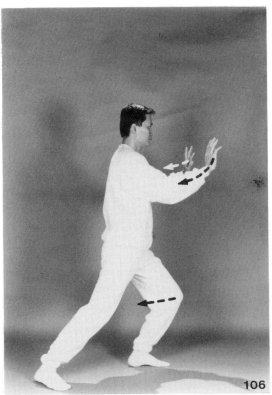

106

(56) Third Waving Hands in the Cloud
San Yun Shou

Movement 1: Shift your weight to the right foot. Turn the torso right 90 degrees, and shift your weight back to the left foot. Lower the left hand to your abdomen with palm inward, and raise your right hand to neck height with palm facing you. Turn your torso gradually right, and shift your weight to the right foot. Continue to turn your torso with both hands right. Shift your weight to the right foot until your left hand and palm are near your abdomen and the right hand, palm down, is near the neck. Assume a ball-holding gesture. Move your left foot close to your right foot. (See photo 107.)

Eyes: Follow your right hand.

Breathing: Inhale.

Mind: Concentrate on the dantian first; then visualize energy coming from the dantian through both arms to both hands and palms.

Self-defense: Use both arms, hands, and palms in front to protect yourself from an attack.

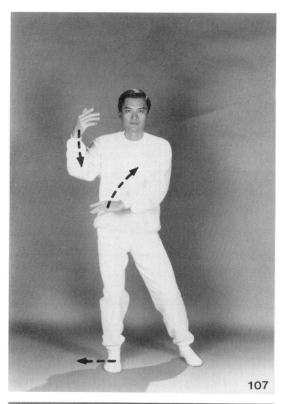

107

Movement 2: Lower your right hand close to your abdomen with palm inward, and raise your left hand to neck height with the palm facing you. Turn your torso gradually left and shift your weight to the left foot slightly. Continue to turn your torso with both hands left. Shift all your weight to the left foot until your right hand, palm up, is near your abdomen and the left hand, palm down, is near your neck. Assume a ball-holding gesture. (See photo 108.)

Eyes: Follow your left hand.

Breathing: Exhale.

Mind: Concentrate on the dantian first; then visualize energy coming from the dantian through both arms to both hands and palms.

Self-defense: Use both arms, hands, and palms in front to protect yourself from attack.

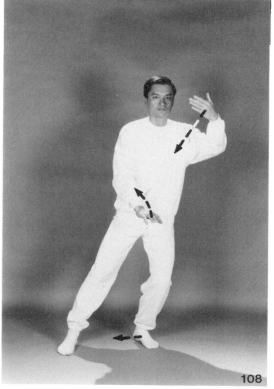

108

(57) Fourth Waving Hands in the Cloud
Si Yun Shou

Movement 1: Move your right foot a step to the right. Lower your left hand to your abdomen with palm facing inward and raise your right hand to neck height with your palm facing you. Turn your torso gradually to the right, and shift your weight to the right foot. Continue to turn your torso along with both hands to the right. Shift all your weight to the right foot until your left hand and palm are near your abdomen and your right hand, palm down, is near your neck. Assume a ball-holding gesture. Move your left foot a step closer to your right foot. (See photo 109.)

Eyes: Follow your right hand.

Breathing: Inhale.

Mind: Concentrate on the dantian first; then visualize energy coming from the dantian through both arms to both hands and palms.

Self-defense: Use both arms, hands, and palms in front to protect yourself from attack.

Movement 2: Lower your right hand to your abdomen with the palm inward, and raise your left hand to neck height with the palm facing you. Turn your torso gradually to the left, and shift your weight to the left foot slightly. Continue to turn your torso together with both hands to the left. Shift all your weight to the left foot until your right hand, palm up, is near your abdomen and your left hand, palm down, is near your neck. Assume a ball-holding gesture. (See photo 110.)

Eyes: Follow your left hand.

Breathing: Exhale.

Mind: Concentrate on the dantian first; then visualize energy coming from the dantian through both arms to both hands and palms.

Self-defense: Use both arms, hands, and palms in front to protect yourself from attack.

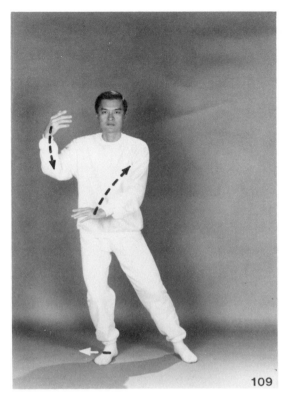

109

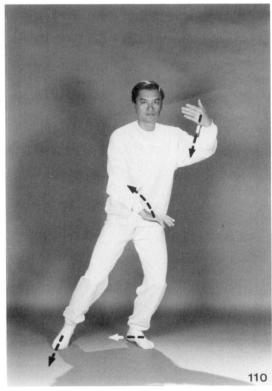

110

(58) Press and Push Hands, Right
You An

Movement: Move your right foot a step forward to your front right side and push out the right palm. (See photo 111.) Bend your left arm and place your left hand inside your right wrist. Turn your torso a little farther right, and press both hands slowly forward with the left palm facing forward, the right hand making a fist, and your right arm rounded. Meanwhile, shift your weight slowly onto your right leg to form a bow step. (See photo 112.)

Eyes: Follow both hands.

Breathing: First inhale, then exhale.

Mind: Concentrate on the dantian first; then visualize energy coming from the dantian through both arms to both hands.

Self-defense: Use both arms and hands to protect yourself and to attack an opponent in front of you.

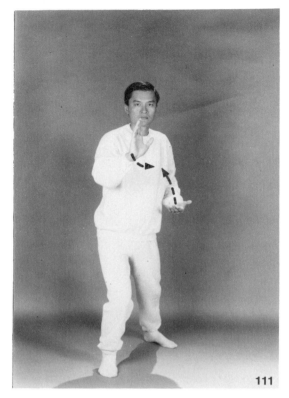

111

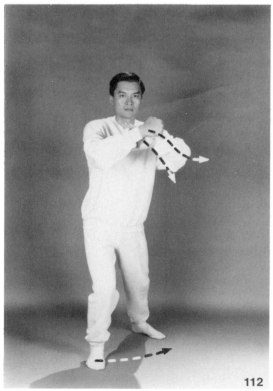

112

(59) Press and Push Hands, Left
Zuo An

Movement: Shift your weight to your left foot first; turn your torso left and move your right foot a step forward to your left side and push out your right palm. (See photo 113.) Bend your right arm and place your right hand inside your left wrist. Turn your torso a little farther left, and press both hands slowly forward with the right palm facing forward and the left hand making a fist, with the left arm rounded. Meanwhile, shift your weight slowly to the left leg to form a bow step. (See photo 114.)

Eyes: Follow both hands.

Breathing: First inhale, then exhale.

Mind: Concentrate on the dantian first; then visualize energy coming from the dantian through both arms to both hands.

Self-defense: Use both arms and hands to protect yourself from attack in front of you and to attack an opponent.

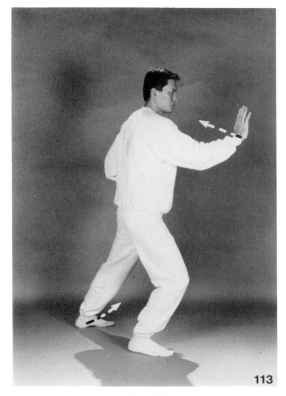

113

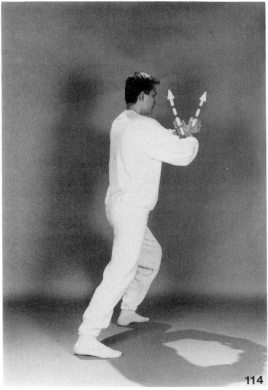

114

(60) Flash the Arm, Left
Zuo Shan Tong Bei

Movement: Shift your weight to your right foot, and move your left foot close to your right foot with the toe touching the ground. Then take a step forward with your left foot to form a bow step, and shift your weight back to your left foot. At the same time, raise your right arm with elbow bent until your hand stops just above your right temple. Turn your palm obliquely upward with your thumb pointing downward. Raise your left hand slightly, and push it forward at nose level with your palm facing forward. (See photo 115.)

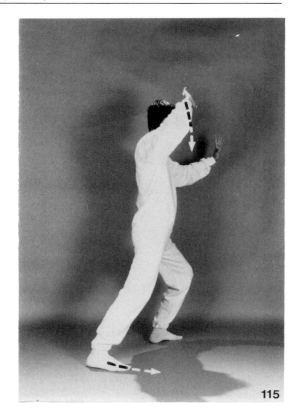

Eyes: Follow your left hand.

Breathing: First inhale, then exhale.

Mind: Concentrate on the dantian first; then visualize energy coming from the dantian through both arms to both hands and palms.

Self-defense: Use your right hand and palm to protect the right side of your head, and use your left hand and palm to attack an opponent in front of you.

Fifth Sequence (61–78)

(61) Press and Push Hands, Right
You An

Movement: Turn your torso to the right and move your right foot a step forward to your right side. Bend your left arm and place your left hand inside your right wrist. Turn your torso a little further right, and press both hands slowly forward with the left palm facing forward, your right hand making a fist, and your left arm rounded. Meanwhile, shift your weight slowly onto the right leg to form a bow step. (See photo 116.)

Eyes: Follow both hands.

Breathing: First inhale, then exhale.

Mind: Concentrate on the dantian first; then visualize energy coming from the dantian through both arms to both hands.

Self-defense: Use both arms and hands to protect yourself and to attack an opponent in front of you.

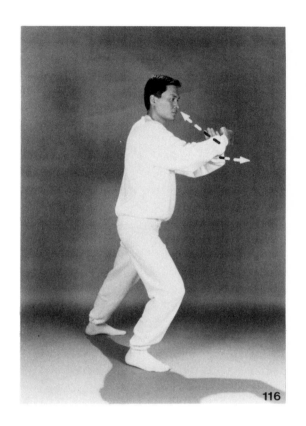

116

(62) Flash the Arm, Right
You Shan Tong Bei

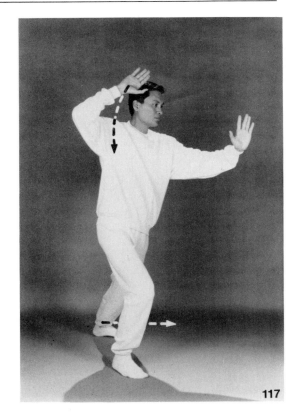

117

Movement: Shift your weight to your left foot, and close your right foot to your left with the toe touching the ground. Then take a step forward with your right foot to form a bow step, and shift your weight back to your right foot. At the same time, raise your right arm with elbow bent until your hand stops just above your right temple. Turn the palm obliquely upward with thumb pointing downward. Raise your left hand slightly, and push it forward at nose level with your palm facing forward. (See photo 117.)

Eyes: Follow your left hand.

Breathing: First inhale, then exhale.

Mind: Concentrate on the dantian first; then visualize energy coming from the dantian through both arms to both hands and palms.

Self-defense: Use your right hand and palm to protect the right side of your head, and use your left hand and palm to attack an opponent in front of you.

(63) Parting the Wild Horse's Mane, Left
Zuo Yei Ma Fen Zong

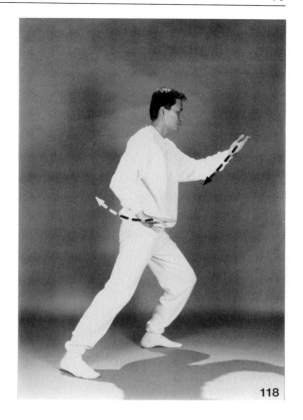

Movement 1: Turn your torso slightly to the right, and move your left foot close to your right foot with the big toe touching the ground. At the same time, move your right hand sideways and up to shoulder level, palm facing downward, and move your left hand back to your right hip with palm facing upward. Assume a ball-holding gesture to the right of your chest, with your right hand on top.

Eyes: Follow your right hand.

Breathing: Inhale.

Mind: Concentrate on the dantian.

Self-defense: Use both hands to protect the right front side of your chest.

Movement 2: Take a step forward with your left foot. Turn the torso a bit farther left, and bend your left leg to form a bow step with your right leg naturally straightened. Shift your weight slowly to the left leg. Meanwhile, push out your rounded left forearm at shoulder level with palm facing inward. Drop your right hand slowly beside the right hip, palm facing downward and fingers pointing forward. (See photo 118.)

Eyes: Follow the left hand.

Breathing: Exhale.

Mind: Visualize energy coming from the dantian through your left arm to your left hand and palm.

Self-defense: Use your left arm, hand, and palm to protect yourself from attack on your left front side.

(64) Turn and Stand on Left Leg
Zhuan Sheng, Zuo Jing Ji Du Li

Movement 1: Shift your weight to the right foot and make a right turn about 120 degrees with your left heel. Shift your weight back to your left foot, and turn a bit farther right. (See photo 119.)

Eyes: Look forward.

Breathing: Inhale.

Mind: Concentrate on the dantian.

Self-defense: Store energy for self-defense.

Movement 2: Move your right hand in front of your chest with your palm facing upward; at the same time, push your left hand outside to your left with palm facing left. Stand on your left foot and move your right foot up with your right heel at the left knee level and push out with your right knee. (See photo 120.)

Eyes: Look forward.

Breathing: Exhale.

Mind: Visualize energy coming from the dantian to both arms, hands, and palms, as well as to your right knee.

Self-defense: Use your right hand to protect your chest and your left hand and palm to attack an opponent on your left side. Use your right foot to protect your left knee and your right knee to attack an opponent in front of you.

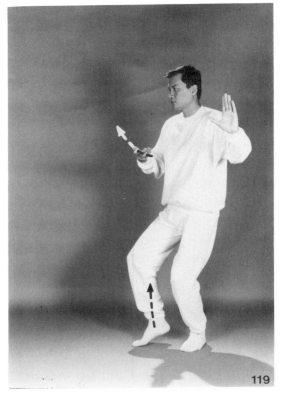

119

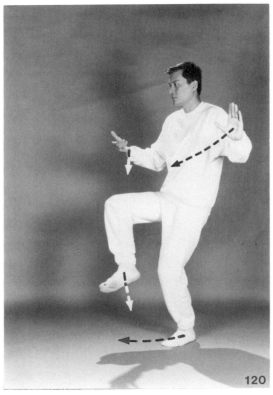

120

(65) Push Down Left Fist
Zuo Zai Chui

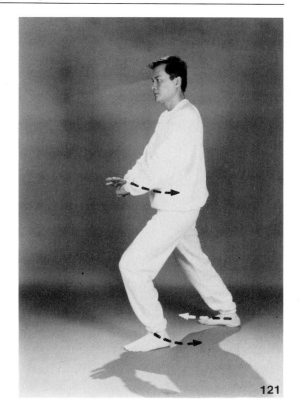

121

Movement 1: Take a step with your right foot in front of you, and shift your weight slightly to your right foot. Move your left foot close to your right foot with the toe touching the ground. At the same time, have both hands circle backwards, outward, forward, and inward until they touch each other with the right palm and left fist in front of your chest.

Eyes: Look forward.

Breathing: Inhale.

Mind: Concentrate on the dantian.

Self-defense: Use both arms and hands, as well as your right palm and left fist, to protect yourself from attack in front of you.

Movement 2: Take a big step with your left foot, and shift your weight to your left. Then push down your right palm with your left fist together with your right palm on top at thigh level. (See photo 121.)

Eyes: Follow both hands.

Breathing: Exhale.

Mind: Visualize energy coming from the dantian through both arms and hands to your right palm and left fist.

Self-defense: Use both arms and hands, and your right palm and left fist, to protect yourself from attack. Use your right foot to kick an opponent in front of you.

(66) Press Right Hand
You An

Movement 1: Shift your weight to your right foot, turn left about 120 degrees, shifting your weight back to your left foot. Move your right foot close to your left foot with the big toe touching the ground; then shift your weight again to your right foot. At this time, the right palm faces up. Move your left hand in front of you. (See photo 122.)

Eyes: Look forward.

Breathing: Inhale.

Mind: Concentrate on the dantian.

Self-defense: Move your body around to protect yourself from an attack from an opponent at your back.

Movement 2: Move your left foot a step forward; then shift your weight to your left foot with your right foot close to your left foot and your right big toe touching the ground. Then move your right foot a step forward with the heel touching the ground first, and shift your weight slightly to your right foot. At the same time, draw your left hand back beside your left hip with palm facing upward, and push your right hand out with palm facing front. (See photo 123.)

Eyes: Follow your right hand.

Breathing: Exhale.

Mind: Visualize energy coming from the dantian through your right arm to your right hand and palm.

Self-defense: Use your left hand and palm to protect your left side from an opponent's attack, and use your right hand and palm to attack an opponent in front of you.

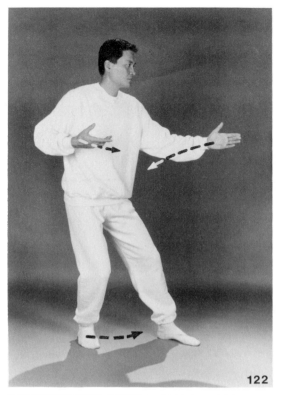

122

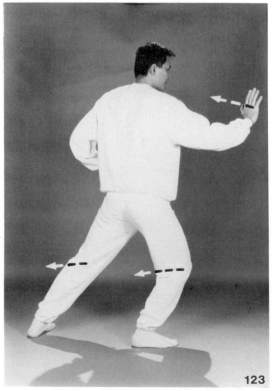

123

(67) Make Fists with Both Hands
Zhua Shuang Chui

Movement: Shift your weight to your left foot, and turn to your left about 90 degrees with your moving right heel. At the same time, change both palms to fists facing upward with your right fist in front of your chest and your left fist beside your left hip. (See photo 124.)

Eyes: Look forward.

Breathing: First inhale, then exhale.

Mind: Concentrate on the dantian first; then visualize energy coming from the dantian through both arms to hands and fists.

Self-defense: Use both arms, hands, and fists to protect yourself from an attack in front of you.

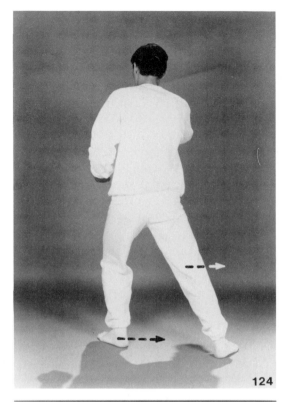

124

(68) Push Down and Stand on One Leg, Left
Zuo Xia Shi, Jing Ji Du Li

Movement 1: Shift your weight to your right foot; pull your left foot back and suspend it by bending your knee with your big toe touching the ground. Form a right-hooked hand, while you turn up your left palm to make an arc upward to the right side until it comes in front of your right shoulder and faces obliquely inward. (See photo 125.) Crouch slowly on your right leg, stretching your left leg outward sideways. Extend your left hand sideways along the inner side of your left leg, palm facing forward. Using your left heel as a pivot, turn the toes of your left foot slightly outward so that they align with the outstretched leg. Turn the toes of your right foot inward while the right leg straightens and the left leg bends. (See photo 126.)

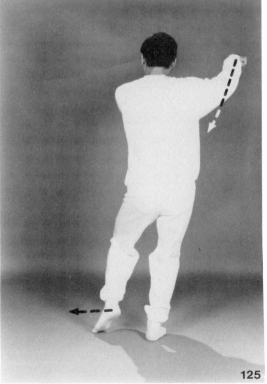

125

continued next page

Eyes: Follow your left hand.

Breathing: Inhale.

Mind: Concentrate on the dantian.

Self-defense: Use your left hand and palm to protect yourself from an attack in front of you.

Movement 2: Shift your weight to your left leg, turn your torso slightly left, and rise slowly in a forward movement. At the same time, continue to extend your left arm forward, with your left palm facing the right side, while you drop your right hand behind the back, with bunched fingertips pointing backwards. Raise your right foot gradually and bend your right knee so that your thigh is level. Then open your right hand, swing it past the outer side of your right leg and upward to the front, until your bent elbow is just above your right knee. Change the palm to a fist. At the same time, change your left palm to a fist in front of your chest to meet your right fist on the outside. (See photo 127.)

Eyes: Follow your left hand first, then your right hand and palm.

Breathing: Exhale.

Mind: Visualize energy coming from the dantian through your right hand and palm to your right knee.

Self-defense: Use your left hand and palm to protect your left side from an opponent's kick, and use your right hand and knee to attack an opponent in front of you.

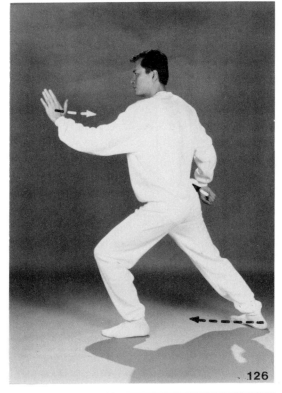

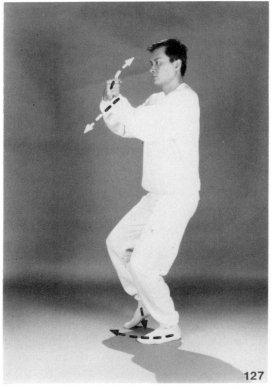

(69) Kick with Left Heel
Zuo Deng Jiao

Movement: Move your right foot down and touch the floor, toe first, and shift your weight to your right foot. Then move your hands away from the center part of your body with your right palm pushing out to the right side and punch your left fist out to your left side. At the same time, kick with your left heel in front of you. (See photo 128.)

Eyes: Look forward.

Breathing: First inhale, then exhale.

Mind: Concentrate on the dantian first; then visualize energy coming from the dantian through both arms to your right palm and left fist, as well as from the dantian to your left foot.

Self-defense: Use your right palm to attack an opponent on your right side, your left fist to attack an opponent on your left side, and your left foot to attack an opponent in front of you.

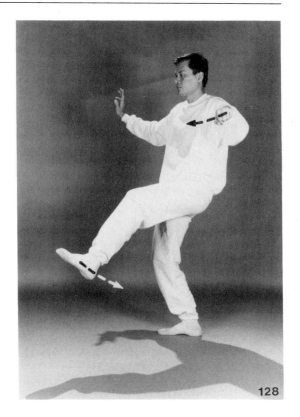

128

(70) Press Right Hand
You An

Movement 1: Move your left foot down and step backwards with your toe touching the ground. Have your right palm facing upward on the right side of your body, and have your left hand circle clockwise in front of your right chest with palm facing downward. Your weight should still be on your right foot. (See photo 129.)

Eyes: Follow both hands.

Breathing: Inhale.

Mind: Concentrate on the dantian.

Self-defense: Use both hands and palms to protect yourself from attack on your front right side.

Movement 2: Shift your weight to your left foot. At the same time, draw your left hand back beside your left hip with palm facing upward, and draw your right hand back in front of your chest. Then push your right hand out again to your right with palm facing right. (See photo 130.)

Eyes: Follow your right hand.

Breathing: Exhale.

Mind: Visualize energy coming from the dantian through your right arm to your right hand and palm.

Self-defense: Use your left hand and palm to protect your left side from an opponent's attack, and use your right hand and palm to attack an opponent in front of you.

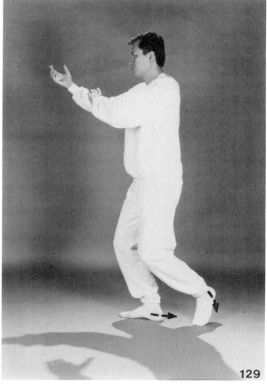

129

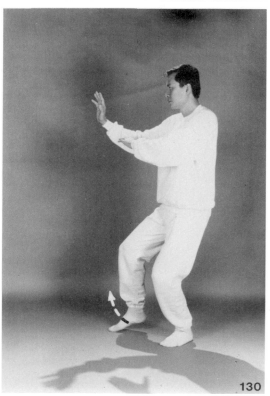

130

(71) Kick with Right Heel and Punch with Left Fist
You Deng Jiao, Zuo Zai Chui

Movement 1: Have your right hand circle counterclockwise until you reach the center of your chest. At the same time, kick with your right heel until you touch your right palm. (See photo 131.)

Eyes: Follow your right hand.

Breathing: Inhale.

Mind: Concentrate on the dantian, and visualize energy coming from the dantian through your right leg to your right foot.

Self-defense: Use your right foot to attack an opponent in front of you.

Movement 2: Move your right foot down and step forward. Shift your weight to your right foot. At the same time, raise your right arm with elbow bent until your hand stops just above your right temple. Then change your right hand to a fist. Raise your left hand slightly, make a fist, and punch it forward at nose level. (See photo 132.)

Eyes: Follow your left hand and fist.

Breathing: Exhale.

Mind: Visualize energy coming from the dantian through both arms to both hands and fists.

Self-defense: Use your right hand and fist to protect your right side, and use your left fist to attack an opponent on your left side.

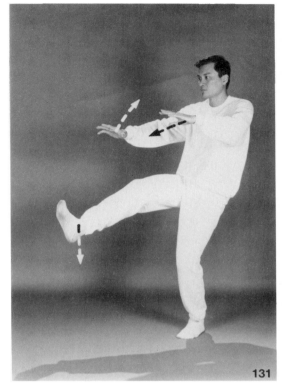

131

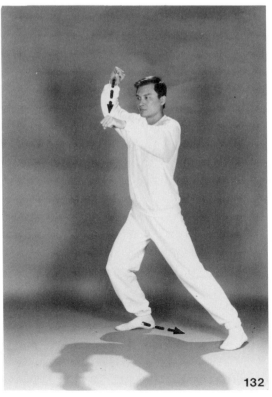

132

(72) Deflect Downward
Ban Lan Chui

Movement: Shift your weight left. Simultaneously have your right hand circle towards the right and downward, and then, with fingers clenched into a fist, move your hand past your abdomen beside your left ribs with knuckles up. (See photo 133.) Thrust right fist upward and forward in front of your chest with knuckles turned down. Lower your left hand to beside your left hip with palm turned downward and fingers pointing forward. At the same time, draw back your right foot, and, without stopping or allowing it to touch the floor, take a step forward with toes turned outward. Shift your weight onto your right foot. (See photo 134.)

Eyes: Follow your right hand and fist.

Breathing: First inhale, then exhale.

Mind: Concentrate on the dantian first; then visualize energy coming from the dantian through your right arm to your right fist.

Self-defense: Use your right fist to attack an opponent on your right front side, and use your left hand to protect your left side.

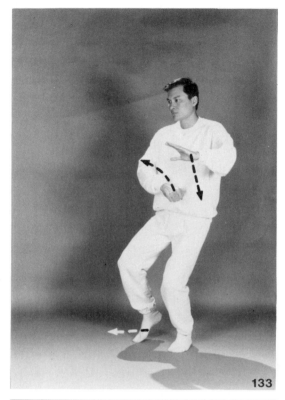

133

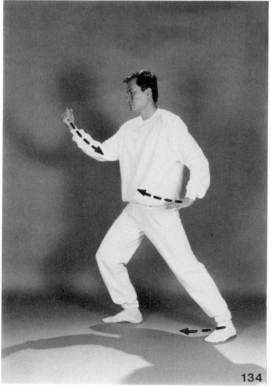

134

(73) Parry and Punch
Zai Chui

Movement: Move your left foot a step forward, and shift your weight slightly to your left foot and bend the left leg to form a bow step. Meanwhile, parry with your left hand, moving up and forward from the left side in a circular movement, with palm turned slightly downward, pulling your right fist in a curve back right, beside your waist with knuckles turned downward. Strike forward at chest level with your right fist, with the back of your hand facing the right side. Pull your left hand back beside your right forearm. (See photos 135 and 136.)

Eyes: Follow your right hand and fist.

Breathing: Inhale first, then exhale.

Mind: Concentrate on the dantian first; then visualize energy coming from the dantian through your right arm to your right fist.

Self-defense: Use your right fist to attack an opponent in front of you.

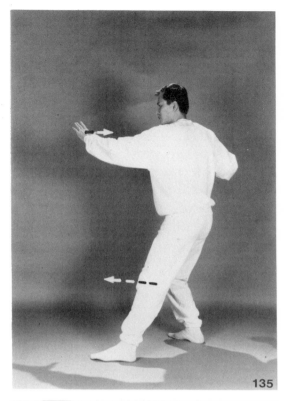

135

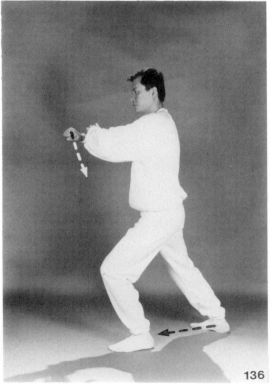

136

(74) Parting the Wild Horse's Mane, Right
You Yei Ma Fen Zong

Movement 1: Turn your torso slightly left, and move your right foot close to your left foot with the big toe touching the ground. At the same time, bring your left hand sideways up to shoulder height with the palm facing downward, and move your right hand back near your left hip with palm facing upward. Assume a ball-holding gesture in front of the left side of your chest, with your left hand on top. (See photo 137.)

Eyes: Follow your left hand.

Breathing: Inhale.

Mind: Concentrate on the dantian.

Self-defense: Use both hands to protect your left front chest.

Movement 2: Take a step forward with your right foot. Turn your torso a bit further right, and bend your right leg to form a bow step with the left leg naturally straightened. Shift your weight slowly to your right leg. Meanwhile, push out the rounded right forearm at shoulder level with palm facing inward. Drop your left hand slowly beside your left hip, palm facing downward and fingers pointing forward. (See photo 138.)

Eyes: Follow the right hand.

Breathing: Exhale.

Mind: Visualize energy coming from the dantian through your right arm to your right hand and palm.

Self-defense: Use your right arm, hand, and palm to protect yourself from an attack on your right front side.

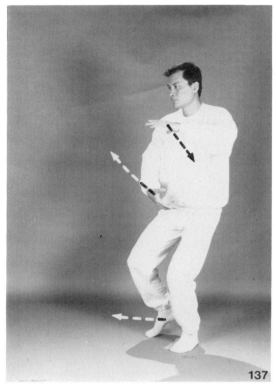

137

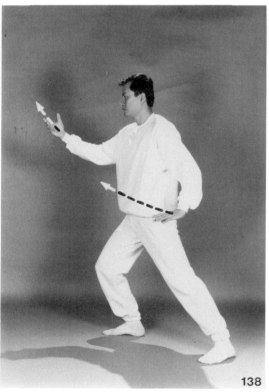

138

(75) Grasp the Bird's Tail, Right
You Lan Jiao Wei

Movement 1: Turn your torso farther right and extend your right hand forward with palm turned down. Bring your left hand upward, palm turning up, until it is below your right forearm. Then turn your torso left while pulling both hands down so that you draw an arc before your abdomen, finishing by extending the left hand sideways at shoulder level, palm up, and by laying the right forearm across the chest, palm turned inward. At the same time, shift your weight to the left foot. (See photos 139 and 140.)

Eyes: Follow your right hand.

Breathing: Inhale.

Mind: Concentrate on the dantian.

Self-defense: Use both arms and hands to grasp an opponent's arm and hand in front of you.

continued next page

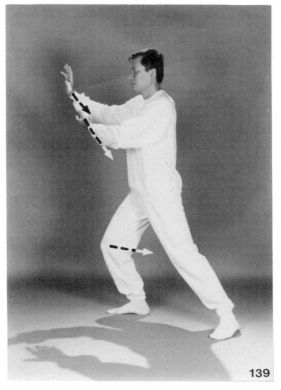

139

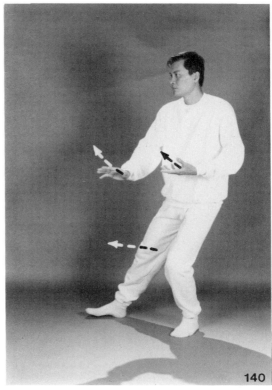

140

Movement 2: Turn your torso slightly right. Bend your left arm and place your left hand inside your right wrist. Turn your torso a little farther right, and press both hands slowly forward with the left palm facing forward and the right palm inward, with the right arm rounded. Meanwhile, slowly shift your weight to your right leg to form a bow step. (See photo 141.)

Eyes: Follow both hands.

Breathing: Exhale.

Mind: Visualize energy coming from the dantian through both arms to your hands and palms.

Self-defense: Use both arms and hands to attack an opponent in front of you.

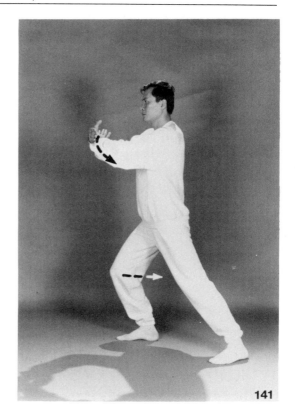

141

(76) Apparent Close
Yu Feng Ci Bi

Movement 1: Turn both palms downward as your left hand passes over your right wrist and moves forward and then left, ending level with your right hand. Separate your hands a shoulder's width apart, and sit back as you shift your weight to the slightly bent left leg. Draw both hands back in front of the abdomen, palms facing slightly downward in front. (See photo 142.)

Eyes: Look forward.

Breathing: Inhale.

Mind: Concentrate on dantian.

Self-defense: Use both arms, hands, and palms to grasp an opponent's shoulders and pull them toward you and down.

Movement 2: Slowly transfer your weight to the right leg while pushing your hands forward and obliquely up, with palms facing forward, until wrists are shoulder height. At the same time, bend your right leg into a bow step. (See photo 143.)

Eyes: Follow both hands.

Breathing: Exhale.

Mind: Visualize energy coming from the dantian through both arms to both hands and palms.

Self-defense: Use both hands and palms to push an opponent's chest away.

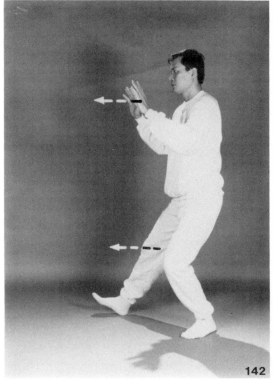

142

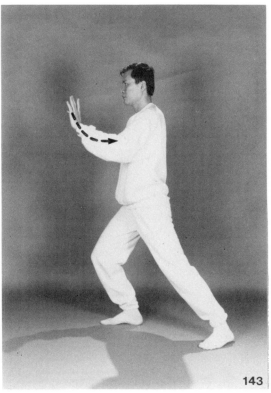

143

(77) Cross Hands
Shi Zi Shou

Movement: Shift your weight to the left foot and turn your body left with the right heel touching the ground. Bend your left knee and sit back. Following the body, turn, and move both hands to your sides in a circular movement at shoulder level, with palms facing forward and elbows slightly bent. Slowly shift your weight to the right leg, and turn the toes of the left foot inward. Then bring your left foot toward the right so that both feet are parallel a shoulder's width apart. Gradually straighten legs; move both hands down and cross them in front of your abdomen. (See photos 144, 145, and 146.)

Eyes: Look forward.

Breathing: Inhale.

Mind: Concentrate on the dantian.

Self-defense: Use both arms and hands to protect your chest.

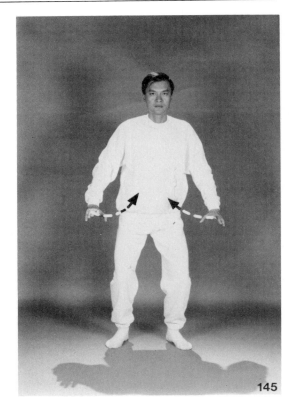

145

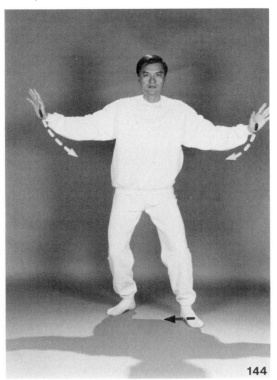

144

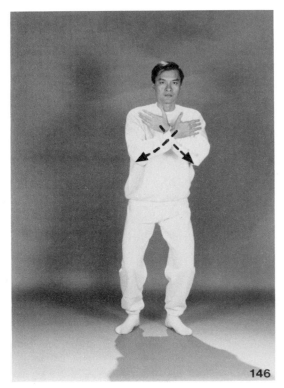

146

(78) Closing Form
Shou Shi

Movement: Turn palms forward and downward while lowering both hands gradually to the side of your hips. (See photo 147.)

Eyes: Look forward.

Breathing: Exhale.

Mind: Visualize energy coming from the dantian through both legs to your feet.

Self-defense: Strengthen both legs and feet by moving the energy down.

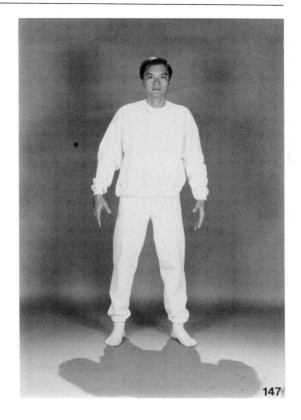

About the Authors

Wei Yue Sun, M.D., attended Sun Yat-sen University of Medical Sciences in Guangzhou, People's Republic of China, where he received his medical degree in 1988. He has practiced both traditional Chinese medicine and Western medicine in China. Dr. Sun has also practiced and taught different styles of tai chi ch'uan for many years in China and, more recently, in the United States.

William Chen, Ph.D., associate professor in the Department of Health Science Education at the University of Florida, is an expert in tai chi ch'uan and a scholar of holistic health. He, like Dr. Sun, has practiced and taught tai chi ch'uan for many years.

The New Style Tai Chi Ch'uan techniques presented in this book are the result of many years of practice and scientific research by Dr. Sun and Dr. Chen.

INDEX